EMMA CANNON'S
TOTAL FERTILITY

EMMA CANNON'S
TOTAL FERTILITY

MACMILLAN

First published 2013 by Macmillan
an imprint of Pan Macmillan, a division of Macmillan Publishers Limited
Pan Macmillan, 20 New Wharf Road, London N1 9RR
Basingstoke and Oxford
Associated companies throughout the world
www.panmacmillan.com

ISBN 978-0-230-76912-0

1 3 5 7 9 8 6 4 2

A CIP catalogue record for this book is available from the British Library.

Designed and set by seagulls.net

Illustrations by Juliet Percival
www.julietpercival.com

Printed and bound by CPI Group (UK) Ltd, Croydon CR0 4YY

This book is intended as a reference volume only, not as a medical manual. The information
given here is designed to help you make informed decisions about your health. It is not
intended as a substitute for any treatment that you may have been prescribed by your doctor.
If you suspect you have a medical problem, we urge you to seek competent medical help.

A Note on Herbal Teas: If pregnant, limit your consumption of herbal teas to a couple of cups
per day. Always speak to your healthcare provider before taking any herbal teas when pregnant.

Visit **www.panmacmillan.com** to read more about all our books and to buy them.
You will also find features, author interviews and news of any author events, and you can
sign up for e-newsletters so that you're always first to hear about our new releases.

For Lily and Violet and the next generation

Health is precious and needs preserving
Fertility is precious and needs preserving

CONTENTS

ACKNOWLEDGEMENTS

I have been lucky enough to have been entrusted by my lovely editor Liz Gough to write this, my second book on my favourite subject: fertility. I am fortunate to have a job that I am deeply passionate about. To be given the chance to write about it and an opportunity to try and change the way we think, even a little, is brilliant beyond belief. So thank you to Liz Gough, Cindy Chan, Jon Butler and everyone at Macmillan for believing in me. Thank you also to Juliet Percival for her beautiful illustrations.

Of course I did not do it alone; thank you to Kate Adams for helping to make sense of my thoughts and chaotic emails and for your patience and calm. You possess qualities I do not have in abundance. Thank you to Violet for being a brilliant travel/writing companion to Kate and me on the train journey through France where time stood still and near disaster was avoided. All in the best of humour, with the aid of some small French beers.

I owe a huge debt to Adrian Lower for painstakingly checking the copy from a medical perspective and writing the brilliant and generous foreword. Thank you to James Nicopoullos from The Lister Fertility Clinic for your contributions. To Michael Dooley for your review and enthusiasm for my work and Bill Smith for your insight into the secret life of the ovaries! Your support and generosity of spirit are greatly appreciated.

To Fiona Arrigo, Henrietta Norton, Kate Freemantle, Michael McIntyre, Uma Dinsmore-Tuli, Tim Weeks, Adriana Giotta, Sheryl Homer, Monika Skrzydlewska, Geeta Nargund, Shideh Pouria, Nicole Pisani and Anna Jones for all your rich and wise contributions.

Thank you to Etta Happe-Thomas, Kate Freemantle, Camilla Fletcher, Laura Hersch and Joanna Ridgeway, for keeping the clinic running smoothly and taking care of all the couples who trust us with their hearts' deepest desires.

Thank you to Claire Norrish, my dear friend and press agent, for always making sure I am shown in my best light and for keeping the press up to date and inspired. To Geraldine Woods for believing in me and being a wise soul.

To Brenda Horton, John Tindall and Great Spirit for being spiritual keepers of my practice. There are some things that happen in life for which a little bit of extra magic is required. I believe there have been times when you have provided just that or you have helped me see what needs to be done in order for progress or change to occur. You understand that as we change and grow as individuals, it resonates for the greater good – that is the true meaning of healing.

To my gorgeous family, Roger, Lily and Violet – thank you for understanding that I am driven by a deep desire and focus to help people become parents. It sometimes means I am absent or distracted. You have my heart even if you do not always have my full focus, especially during book editing!

Lastly, to my lovely readers and patients. I owe you the biggest debt of gratitude for sharing your hopes and dreams with me and for believing in my approach. I learn from your strength and am inspired by your bravery every day. Thank you for the many letters and emails I receive and for all the feedback you have given me, either from your consultations with me or from reading my books or articles. I am blessed.

FOREWORD

Emma Cannon has produced another first-class book. This time the emphasis is very much on preservation of fertility – that precious gift that none of us value until it is too late and it is gone. Through this book Emma provides important information for all women about some of the influences they will encounter during their lives that may impact on their fertility and how they can minimize the negative effects and promote the positives.

The messages are important and relevant for all women and Emma provides useful and concrete advice for those who find themselves struggling to start their families rather later in life – because nobody told them that their fertility was a finite resource.

Through practical advice based on the fundamental principles of Chinese Medicine Emma is able to provide a road map to help women find their way through the difficult journey to motherhood when the obstacles seem stacked against them. Her approach promotes health and wellbeing and whilst many of her clients may be panicking that their biological clock is running out of time, she emphasizes the importance of getting life and the body back in harmony and this takes time. Following this investment of time and effort many women will conceive spontaneously; others are better prepared to respond to the interventions of conventional practitioners.

Emma Cannon is a powerful healer with a hugely positive aura who has a significant impact on all those who come into contact with her, whether they be clients or colleagues. She possesses great wisdom and understanding, and with her roots in Eastern Medicine she has developed a very sophisticated understanding of the problems of fertility and has established a network of complementary and conventional medical practitioners who share her passion for an integrated approach; together they provide a remarkable synthesis of care. This holistic approach to fertility is encapsulated in this book. Emma writes very clearly and her books are easy to read and full of practical tips and messages that empower her patients, providing a structure and framework that they can embrace and enabling them to take personal responsibility and gain positively from a sense of practical involvement in their care.

This book is a first step in the battle against declining fertility.

Mr Adrian Lower FRCOG
Consultant Gynaecologist and Fertility Specialist
London, April 2013

INTRODUCTION

Fertility is one of the major health and wellbeing issues for modern women. Whether it's women in their twenties with gynaecological issues or problems with their menstrual cycle, those in their early thirties looking ahead and worrying whether they will be able to have children when the right time comes, the growing numbers of women who have experienced at least one miscarriage, or women simply needing clear, warm and supportive advice while trying for a baby, fertility is central to women's health and yet so often ignored or medicalized to the point where we don't give nature enough of a chance.

As a specialist in integrated health and fertility for nearly twenty years, my aim is to cut through all the statistics and offer you clear advice and encouragement on your own unique fertility journey. I want to equip you with a guide that answers all those nagging questions you may have and don't know who to ask. Questions such as: 'How can I get a sense of my fertility?' 'Can I preserve my fertility?' 'When exactly should we be having sex?' 'Does my diet really matter?' or 'Does stress lower my chances of conceiving?'

In my practice I see women with a huge variety of reasons for wanting support with their fertility. Some women want to raise their health levels prior to conceiving; many are worried they might struggle to get pregnant; others have been trying for many months without success but are being offered no help or support from anywhere else. Couples also come to see me for extra support through IVF and other treatments, asking about the things they can do to help themselves. In my experience, couples really want guidance, and so I am here to offer simple, practical advice to help you through the minefield that can be the fertility journey.

We are all individual in the way we deal with things in our lives. My aim is that this book should be a friendly and helpful guide to support you along the way, no matter what stage you are at along the path to becoming parents. I am often amazed by the things that aren't covered in other books or online. There is so little about sex in fertility books, and yet of course it is a pretty important part of the whole having-a-baby process! I also read very little about how power of the mind can affect fertility, while I know from twenty years of experience that our attitude and approach to fertility is often one of the most important factors.

I don't need to convince women that our bodies go through physical changes each and every monthly cycle. I can easily show you how our fertility will improve if we nourish rather than try to ignore these changes. For so many women nowadays, an awareness of fertility preservation is essential, as not all of us are ready to have a baby in our twenties: we may be putting our careers first, or we may not be with the right partner. It is something women often think about but have little knowledge of – other than the lovely statistic declaring that your fertility falls off a cliff on or around your thirty-fifth birthday. The reality is that, yes, our chances of conception do decrease as we age, but it is also the case that every woman is an individual and there is much we can do to look after our fertility and our overall health. I want you to benefit from the wisdom I can share. I will show you what you can do to help preserve your fertility – and your overall health – and optimize your fertile time.

PART ONE
YOUR FERTILITY

My approach is to help patients to become parents from a place of health and balance. I do this by offering a combination of the best of all approaches: from general wellbeing methods, lifestyle changes, correct fertility awareness and acupuncture through to using the most advanced medical techniques available.

I see couples from all walks of life. Many are hardworking couples, some of whom are used to achieving, and it can come as quite a shock if they don't fall pregnant when they expect to. Often this will be the first failure they have experienced. Of course, it isn't a failure: it is quite normal for conception to take a little while, especially when you factor in all the modern-day pressures that affect all of us.

Sometimes a consultation with a couple is just about reassuring them that they are normal and giving some general information about how they might improve their health and diet and be more fertility aware. Sometimes it is much more involved, and couples may need medical intervention. In each case I always work with a team of experts, the best in their field, people who I know and trust. Although my medical colleagues are trained in an entirely different way to me, we have the same aim: to help couples achieve healthy pregnancies and healthy babies.

When I sit with a couple for the first time, I always ask myself the same questions:

- How can I help to make their bodies work optimally to aid conception? This will, of course, depend on how far their bodies have deviated from normal functioning.
- How can I preserve their fertility?
- What can they do to help themselves?

The aim of this book is to help you answer these questions yourself, as well as encourage you to seek help when you feel you have done as much as you can to help yourself.

HOW THE BOOK WORKS

In the first half of the book I offer information on the various complementary methods you can use to enhance your fertility, including lots of fertility-boosting recipes to enjoy throughout the month, advice on fertility-boosting exercise, plus all the practical and emotional support I offer my patients during any treatments, information on what to expect from any tests you might need, and also a chapter on charting your cycle that will give you an amazing sense of fertility awareness. Look out for the 'toolbox' sections: these focus on the practical things you can do to make a difference to your fertility. The latter half of the book looks at ways to support assisted reproductive techniques, including IVF, as well as advice on managing common fertility conditions. At the end of the book you will find a glossary of terms used, along with information on the various complementary treatments I recommend throughout. My hope is that whatever stage of the fertility journey you are at, even if you are thinking of having a family in the future, there will be something useful for you in these pages.

CHAPTER ONE
A NEW APPROACH TO FERTILITY

I want to explain a little about Chinese medicine here because I find it so helpful to the fertility journey. My work as an acupuncturist comprises a great deal more than the physical process of putting needles into specific points on the body. I have included a more detailed list of complementary treatments that are helpful for fertility at the back of the book (see page 253).

For those of you who are unfamiliar with the practice, Chinese medicine is a completely holistic philosophy that involves not only the body but also the mind. It looks at how we all manage stress; what we eat and drink, as well as when, where and how we eat; the balance between exercise and rest; and our relationships and environments at home and at work. In Chinese medicine the menstrual cycle is seen as the foundation of health for women, as it reveals so much about both our fertility and our general wellbeing.

My experience has shown me that different systems of medicine have their own strengths and weaknesses. Put Chinese medicine and Western medicine together and you have a combination that I have seen help so many people, especially in the field of fertility. For example, IVF treatment is one of the biggest breakthroughs in modern medicine, but it simply cannot address all the issues associated with infertility and subfertility. Of course, the doctors, the experts in Western medicine, are concentrating on the 'big shift', i.e. stimulating the ovaries, collecting the eggs and putting them together with the sperm to make the embryos. Meanwhile, through my acupuncture work, and experience in offering patients other complementary therapies, I am there in the background doing what I like to call the 'fine tuning' using the principles of Chinese medicine – so I will gently increase the patient's blood flow to her follicles and womb lining, help calm her mind, and, post-transfer, help to stop contractions and aid implantation. This is an example, in my view, of integrated medicine at its very best.

THE BENEFITS OF ACUPUNCTURE FOR FERTILITY

- Optimizes the natural menstrual cycle
- Manages menstrual symptoms
- Prepares couples for IVF
- Supports couples through IVF cycle-receptiveness
- Calms the mind
- Manages symptoms of ovarian hyperstimulation syndrome (OHSS)
- Helps restore good blood flow after surgery (for example, after surgery to remove fibroids or treat uterine scarring and during IVF)
- Helps with endometrium problems
- Helps with ovulation problems, especially anovulation (lack of ovulation)

DIFFERENTIAL DIAGNOSIS

I do not want to blind you with too much unfamiliar language in this book, because what I aim to do every day is to help patients connect with their own body and health. But there is one main concept that underpins the way that I practise and resonates most with the patients, and that is 'differential diagnosis'. The basic idea is that rather than taking a one-size-fits-all approach to conditions, the treatment should depend on the needs of the individual, which are influenced by their constitution (what I call Jing), their lifestyle and environment, and also their mind and emotions.

When a patient comes to me with an existing condition, like endometriosis for example, I won't automatically treat her in the same way as another patient with the same condition. We are all different and each condition manifests itself differently in each person based on their internal environment, and it is that environment that I am trying to change and that we are going to work on in this book.

I have included only the key concepts of Chinese medicine that I use with patients. I find that rather than feeling blinded by jargon, people actually really like these explanations because they make so much sense. At the back of the book, I have also included basic treatment options for each of these principles, which I will refer to during the course of the book.

KEY PRINCIPLES OF CHINESE MEDICINE

Blood is a term used a great deal in Chinese medicine and in particular in relation to fertility. We consider the quality of Blood during menstruation, and so will look at ways to 'build' the Blood through diet and lifestyle (as well as acupuncture) and also 'move' the Blood at the right times of the month. Blood ensures that our endometrium (the lining of the uterus) is well nourished and welcoming to an embryo. It is helpful for patients to develop a healthier cycle that ebbs and flows with regularity and without the extremes of terrible pain or wild mood swings. So many women are running on empty, under-resting and perhaps under-eating.

In Chinese medicine we see a strong connection between the Heart and the Womb. What nourishes the Heart nourishes the Womb. In Western medicine the links between stress and how it affects the menstrual cycle are now becoming more widely recognized and accepted. In my experience, the mind and emotions are absolutely key to fertility, with the ability to help when strong and hinder when weak.

Yin and Yang are well-known Chinese-medicine terms, and it won't come as a surprise that working on the balance of traditionally female and male energies in the body is an important part of how we approach fertility, and in particular the menstrual cycle. We consider the first half of the cycle, pre-ovulation (follicular), to be the Yin phases, which build gently and then give way to the more energetic Yang phases of ovulation and post-ovulation (luteal). The language might be slightly different, but there are clear parallels with how we see hormones acting during the cycle and also the changes in body temperature. Yin represents the potential, which is when oestrogen gently builds towards ovulation. And then Yang represents the incubation phase (and also the sperm in conception), when progesterone and warmth take over.

Qi, pronounced 'chee', is that feeling of energy that runs through us. It is our sense of vitality, or sometimes the lack of it when we are feeling out of sorts or when we are ill. When I work with a patient, I try to detect whether their Qi is flowing well and smoothly, is lacking, or perhaps a bit stuck – or as we say 'Stagnant' (when they are irritable or emotionally a bit unstable). I will show you how to nourish your Qi at the optimum times in the middle of your menstrual cycle and also allow it to rest and replenish at other times, like during your period, rather than go hell for leather all month long which so often leads to a feeling of burnout.

Heat and Cold are two of the main 'climates' I will detect in a patient's body, and these are often manifested in their emotions. As in everything, we are looking to create a balance, and this is important in relation to the menstrual cycle in particular. Too much Heat early on in the cycle and Yin doesn't get a chance to build nice and gently; too much Cold later on and we don't create that lovely incubating environment needed post-ovulation. When I see a patient is out of balance I advise them to include warming or cooling foods in their diet as needed, and in the section In the Fertility Kitchen (see page 54) I have included lots of recipes that help to encourage the right climate at the right time of the month.

Damp is something I am often on the lookout for with patients because the climate here in the UK and also our diet (too much sugar, dairy and alcohol) can be quite Dampening in the body. Exposure to STDs or infection can also create and leave a legacy of Dampness in the body. In fertility, Damp can inhibit the smooth passage of the egg through the Fallopian tubes. In some cases it can form fluid-filled cysts on the ovaries and be a factor in preventing an egg from being released. The easiest way to describe Damp is to think of when you are bloated with water retention: the body is holding on to excess water and disrupting the internal climate, making it waterlogged (and often Stagnant).

Jing represents our constitutional health: what is in our genes and also passed down to us in terms of how healthy our parents were when they had us. So this affects our general state of health and also offers us indicators of conditions to which we might be more susceptible. You know how some people seem to be 'as strong as an ox'? In terms of fertility, I think of Jing as being a bit like 'asking your mum' – she and the other women in your family always hold so much valuable information. When looking after our health, we need to combine an understanding of our Jing with how we live day to day: our lifestyle, our diet and the way we look after our emotions. In terms of optimum fertility, and indeed optimum health, that is always the key.

I tend to use the word Stagnation a great deal, because it is a big issue in fertility. Emotionally we can become Stagnant when life's frustrations build up. Everyday things like spilling the contents of the dustbin over yourself (when you'd asked your partner to empty it three times), being stuck in a traffic jam or losing your car keys and getting irrationally cross about it – all these are signs of Stagnation. Or it can be the frustration of not getting where you want to in life and feeling that your vision has been thwarted. I see it often in my patients: the signs that point to Stagnation for me are the deep sigh, the line between the eyebrows, irregular periods or bowel movements.

Over time this Stagnation can begin to affect the organs of the pelvic cavity, inhibit the Fallopian tubes and interrupt the release of an egg. Eventually Stagnant energy can become Stagnant Blood – a factor in cysts, endometriosis, fibroids and so on. So a huge part of my job is to keep energy moving well around the body. Exercise, acupuncture, breathing techniques and abdominal massage are all good ways to achieve this, alongside a generally healthy lifestyle.

A great deal to do with fertility relies on 'transport' and movement. The egg must be released and travel down the Fallopian tube; the sperm must reach the egg; the fertilized egg needs to find its way to implanting in the endometrium. This is why it's so important to have good 'flow': it means a good transport system and a smooth journey for your precious fertilized egg!

CHAPTER TWO
THE FERTILE WOMAN

Our ability to preserve our health is one of the most important strands of the field of medicine I work in. In this chapter I want to describe exactly how our fertility works and some of the ways you can enhance and protect fertility health, from being aware of your menstrual cycle and your gynaecological health to generating and safeguarding life and fertility from within.

PROTECTING YOUR FERTILITY

Your current health and fertility is made up of several factors: the genes you inherited from your parents; illnesses, STDs, accidents, lifestyle choices; your emotional picture; and environmental factors like the level of endocrine disruptors you have been exposed to (including the type of work you have done). So if your parents were non-drinking, non-smoking twenty-year-olds when they had you and you have lived like a nun your whole life without illness or accident, you probably have no need for this book. But if, like most of us, you have drunk from the cup of life, burnt the candle at both ends from time to time and stayed up to see the sun rise on more than one occasion, then a little refining and fine-tuning may be of great benefit.

You need to take care to understand your menstrual cycle and your gynaecology, protect yourself from STDs, give up smoking (yes, that is a must, I am afraid), take adequate rest, eat a regular and balanced diet, have one drink but never three (!) and be as healthy as possible. Sound boring? It doesn't have to be. It is possible to make healthy changes and embrace the earth mother in you without getting rid of all the rock and roll – and that is what I intend to show you in this book. We will make simple changes together with joy in our hearts because you will feel the best you have in years.

HEALTH IN BALANCE

Everything I do as a practitioner aims to help bring my patients back into balance. And I think it makes sense to every one of us that our fertility really is all about balance. When all is well with our fertility, there are so many amazing things that happen as a result. Of course there is the meeting of the sperm with the egg for conception, but before that there is an ebb and flow of hormones that causes the release of an egg during each monthly cycle and creates a fertile environment for implantation: cooling and moist in the build-up to the release; warm and receptive in the second half of the cycle. When our energy is in a good balance, neither Stagnant nor burnt out (Deficient), we encourage these processes that are going on in our bodies. When our minds are relaxed and focused, so too are our bodies. We eat well, not too much but also not too little. We energize ourselves with exercise while taking a little time to rest our frantic minds.

Creating a balance within the body is my purpose, as I hope to convey throughout this book. Whether you are looking to get pregnant right now, you wish to preserve your fertility for the future, or you feel you might need some kind of medical help, the aim is actually always the same. And the first step towards enhancing your fertility is to become your own healer; after all, you know your body better than anyone else and I truly believe 'Healing comes from within'.

MENSTRUAL CYCLE AWARENESS

Our menstrual cycles tell us so much about our fertility, and our general wellbeing too. It's not something we tend to talk about, other than to complain of irritability, pain or exhaustion at certain times of the month. Through diet and lifestyle you can actually address all of these more negative signs, and by building an awareness of your cycle you can get to know your fertility health. In Chapter 8 I show you how to chart and interpret your menstrual cycle. You will understand the key signs of ovulation, whether you are producing the vital fertile mucus around that time, how regular your periods are, whether you are bleeding too little or too much, and whether there are lifestyle adjustments you can make at certain times of the month to improve things. Many patients who follow the lifestyle advice included in this book often come to me just a few months later reporting pain-free periods and feeling that everything is generally more regular and balanced on both the physical and emotional side of things. And of course many happily report a pregnancy.

It's interesting that the key signals I look for run in parallel with the Western description of how the hormones rise and fall during the cycle, stimulating a number of complex and crucial events, mainly menstruation and ovulation. The first half of the cycle is dominated by oestrogen, related to stimulating follicle growth, egg development and building up of fertile mucus towards ovulation. And then in the second half, progesterone takes over, combined with a definite rise in temperature (see page 150 for more about charting your BBT, or body basal temperature). I describe the first half of the cycle as the Yin phase, and focus very much on how the follicles and egg develop, how important fertile mucus is and the gentle build-up of the lining of the uterus. And I describe the second half as the Yang phase, which is very focused on action and warmth: the act of releasing the egg, when our mind needs to be calm and our energy flowing, and then warming the Womb, ready to be an incubator.

Encouraging a natural ebb and flow of hormones is the aim of both conventional and complementary approaches to conception, which is why I favour the integrated route so much – in my experience it offers women the best of both worlds.

Throughout the cycle, the key messages I convey to my patients correspond with these four phases:

Phase 1: During your period

Moving the Blood. It is so important to fully shed the endometrium (the lining of the uterus) each cycle. This allows the new lining to start from scratch, which then becomes very helpful post-ovulation in creating the perfect environment for a fertilized egg.

Phase 2: Follicular

Building or nourishing the Blood. Similarly, building the Blood relates to the quality of the lining of the uterus, and also the quality of the fertile mucus and the ovaries, and in turn the follicles and the developing egg.

Phase 3: Ovulation

Calming the mind. Emotional upset can play havoc with hormones and the menstrual cycle. We pay particular attention to the mind around ovulation, as stress can even prevent ovulation in some cases. Later in the cycle, this emotional upset is more noticeable, as it often shows in symptoms of PMS.

Phase 4: Luteal

Warming the Womb. Warmth during the period and in the second half of the cycle is essential. I am like a broken record with my patients when I tell them not to swim during their period or eat Cold energy foods like ice cream or bananas! Remember, this is the incubation phase.

GYNAECOLOGICAL HEALTH AWARENESS

The female genital tract comprises the vulva, vagina, cervix, Fallopian tubes and ovaries. Engaging in your gynaecological health is essential for fertility and for your overall health. If, for example, there is a history of fibroids or ovarian cysts in your family, it is a good idea to talk to your doctor sooner rather than later so that they can keep an eye on things and keep you up to

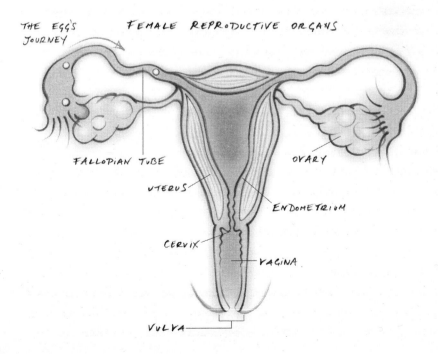

THE EGG'S JOURNEY

FEMALE REPRODUCTIVE ORGANS

FALLOPIAN TUBE

OVARY

UTERUS

ENDOMETRIUM

CERVIX

VAGINA

VULVA

date on your medical options. Likewise, it is good to be aware of conditions such as polycystic ovary syndrome (PCOS), premature ovarian failure (page 31), Asherman's syndrome (page 17) and endometriosis (see below), as these are conditions that can affect fertility but equally can be helped a great deal through treatment or in some cases diet and lifestyle. (In Part 3 I will explain assisted conception and fertility treatments in detail, and also everything you can do yourself during these treatments to aid the process.) Here are some of the gynaecological issues that often affect a woman's fertility.

- The endometrium lines the uterus and becomes thicker towards the end of the menstrual cycle to provide the right environment for the fertilized egg. If fertilization doesn't occur, the top layer breaks down and so we have our period. Endometriosis is a condition in which cells that should live inside the uterus migrate to other areas of the body, most commonly in the lower part of the pelvis including the ovaries and Fallopian tubes. They might also migrate to the bladder or rectum, or even to the small intestine, kidneys or stomach. If left to develop, these patches or lesions can lead to intense pelvic pain and affect fertility (see pages 191–4).

- Pelvic inflammatory disease (PID) can occur following an infection of the reproductive organs. Salpingitis is an infection of the Fallopian tubes that may cause an obstruction to the free passage of sperm through the tubes. Ureaplasma, candida (see page 180) and chlamydia (see page 22) can be to blame for chronic PID. Although it can usually be treated with antibiotics, some cases can be stubborn. I find that lifestyle adjustments, acupuncture and herbs can be helpful.

- Every month an egg is released from one of the ovaries and travels down into the Fallopian tubes, where it may be fertilized, and on into the uterus. As you get to know your menstrual cycle (see pages 145–86) you will have a good indication of whether or not you are ovulating regularly. Some women ovulate infrequently (oligomenorrhoea) or not at all (amenorrhoea; see page 162). This is usually due to resistant ovaries or premature ovarian failure.

- Polycystic ovary syndrome (PCOS) is a hormone-related condition where small, underdeveloped follicles grow on the ovaries (see pages 194–7). Symptoms include irregular or absent periods, acne, weight gain and hair growth on the face or chest (or male pattern baldness). If left unmanaged, it can cause problems with fertility, as ovulation is less likely to occur.

- Fibroids are lumps that form for no apparent reason in the wall of the uterus. In some women they cause heavy menstrual bleeding and can be painful, especially during pregnancy. They can also cause pain during intercourse, urinary trouble, such as the frequent need to urinate, or infections (see pages 197–9). They can be removed if necessary, but research suggests that a healthy balanced diet and lifestyle will go a long way to preventing them from causing serious problems, especially if they are detected early.

- Ovarian cysts are small fluid-filled sacs that grow on the ovaries and usually clear up within a couple of months. They don't tend to affect fertility directly, but they can be an indicator of the type of hormone inbalances that might be a problem.

- Asherman's syndrome is an often under-diagnosed condition that can affect a woman's fertility without her knowing. This is when there is scarring in the uterus, usually from a previous procedure, for example a sharp curettage (scraping) following miscarriage or to remove the placenta after giving birth, a Caesarian section or surgery to remove fibroids or polyps. (Polyps may inhibit embryo implantation, impair sperm transport or cause abnormal menstrual bleeding, so it may be advisable to remove them in infertile women or those commencing fertility treatment.) The trauma to the endometrial lining triggers the normal healing process, which can lead to scarring that may affect fertility. The only real symptoms are an absence of or scanty periods, but with pain. If you have had a procedure in the past and experience these symptoms, it may well be worth investigating as Asherman's is often missed and can be treated by an experienced surgeon. A hysteroscopy or hysterosalpingogram are the most reliable methods for diagnosis (see page 208). I believe acupuncture and herbal medicine have an important role to play post-operatively in helping return the endometrium to its normal function and establish a healthy blood flow to the ovaries and endometrium.

- A retroverted uterus is where the uterus tilts backwards so that the cervix points upwards; some people believe this may make it hard for the sperm to travel through the cervix to the uterus. There is no medical evidence to support this. A retroverted uterus can make an embryo transfer a little tricky, however.

- Premature ovarian failure is otherwise known as early menopause and early signs can include irregular or missed periods, vaginal dryness and hot flushes. In rare cases this can reverse itself. It is important to be aware of any signs early, so that you can see a fertility specialist and explore your options (see page 32).

All these conditions seem to be on the increase, partly due to better diagnostics and partly, I suspect, to environmental factors at play.

ASK YOUR MUM

Our relationship with our mothers is probably the most intense relationship we experience, in one way or another, even in absence. Our mother literally gives us life. Every woman contains within her the essence of her mother, her grandmother, great-grandmother and every woman that has gone before her. The mother–daughter relationship therefore contains the emotional and physical building blocks for life. Our mother has such a profound influence on our present and future health. For better or for worse, we are our mothers' daughters.

So how did mothers get so overlooked in the fertility story? Looking through many books on the subject, they barely get a mention. Perhaps a reliance on medicine and science and testing has overtaken intuition. But this is science – biologically we are likely to suffer from similar conditions to our mothers. The women in your family are a huge source of information that can offer an opportunity to optimize your fertility.

When thinking about your own fertility, if you are lucky enough to still have your mother around, I suggest sitting down and talking to her about these things. If you don't have a good relationship with your mother or she is no longer in your life, I hope you will be able to talk to other women in your family. I know I am lucky to be one of five girls, so we always openly discussed these issues. If my mum didn't fill me in, my sisters did. I knew everything about my own birth and my mother's fertility and that of my sisters long before I had my own children – maybe that is why I find this whole subject so incredible. But I have learnt, to my surprise, that many families do not discuss this sort of thing at all. Many girls receive precious little guidance on female health and sexuality. I think it's such a shame. We owe it to our children to be open and honest about health, and particularly periods and sex. It's never too late to start being open; some of our parents were born into a very different world, so perhaps they considered it self-indulgent to talk about their health. But you can change that; maybe your mum will appreciate your interest in your health heritage. And you could be doing yourself the biggest favour by learning some vital information that might prevent history from repeating itself.

Here are some good questions to ask your mum:

- What age was your mother when she had you? In terms of inherited constitution, the younger your mum was when she had you, the better for your inherited fertility potential.
- How was her health and how was the pregnancy, birth and the postnatal period? If she was unwell or traumatized during pregnancy, labour or postnatally, this could have had an impact on your constitution.
- Did she smoke or have a problem with drink or drugs? This tells you about her state of health while pregnant. All of these aspects can affect the health of the foetus (i.e. you).

- Did she suffer from emotional problems – at any time but particularly post-birth? This may tell you something about the emotional environment you were born into.
- Did she have gynaecological issues such as fibroids? There is evidence of some hereditary predisposition to certain conditions (see page 21).
- Did she have any miscarriages? These might have left her depleted, or it may indicate an inherited condition like a clotting disorder or thyroid problem (see page 199).
- Did she have long periods between the birth of her children? This may indicate she struggled to conceive, although of course it could be down to choice or male fertility issues.
- Did she have thyroid problems? Again, these can be hereditary.
- Did anyone in the family have blood clotting disorders? These can lead to implantation problems.
- Did anyone suffer from autoimmune conditions? Immunology is now considered a factor in fertility (see page 220).
- Did she go through early menopause? This is an important consideration when it comes to age and fertility, i.e. your ovarian reserve (see page 31).[11]

I remember an interesting case of a woman whose mother went through the menopause at forty, and when I asked about the family history there were four generations of only children. They were also Irish Catholics, who tend to have many children as they do not use contraception. So this might be a clue to the fertility of the women in this family line, since without contraception it is likely there would have been more children.

HOW YOUR MOTHER SHAPED YOU

When I set out to write this book, I wanted to let women know just how much we can affect our fertility. We are not powerless. To be warned is to be armed, and if you know your mum had fibroids in her thirties, for example, that is powerful knowledge. Equally, ask yourself what emotional tendencies she may have passed on to you. This is not for the purpose of judging what is 'good' or 'bad', but simply to get to know ourselves better. It is my belief that connecting with your own mother and understanding her physical and emotional health will go some way to bringing you closer to becoming a mother yourself.

Of course, the factors that may have affected your mum won't automatically affect you; but it is interesting to assess the general family background and look for clues. Sometimes I will ask a patient about her relationship with her mother and it will really open up the dialogue to reveal deeply held beliefs about themselves, their health and even their fertility. Among the older women I see, many of these women rightly or wrongly felt a pressure from their mothers, society or themselves to achieve and do things the previous generation of women never had the chance to do. Some women tell me how lucky they feel to have great jobs and opportunities, but that there is a huge part of them that would like the chance to 'just be a mum'. There is a guilt that goes with this, as if somehow that's not enough, or they should feel lucky to be able to do what their mothers couldn't. We need to realize that our life and our health is in one sense what we inherit, but it's also about the choices we make and how we choose to live our lives, both physically and emotionally. We have to realize that we are often masters of our own destiny. As women, one of the most healing and compassionate things we can do is forgive: we can forgive our mothers their shortcomings, realize our own and move forward with compassion, looking forward to a future that belongs to us and our children. We come from a very different world and our children are being born into and creating a different world to ours.

THE IMPACT OF STDs

One of the two most common causes of female fertility problems is blockages in or damage to the Fallopian tubes. An untreated chlamydia infection, for example, can develop into pelvic inflammatory disease, blocking the Fallopian tubes. It is therefore crucial to take very good care of your sexual health and seek medical help if there is any chance that you may have picked up an infection. Sexually active people should be regularly screened for both bacterial infections and STDs.

Chlamydia, which is estimated to affect up to 10 per cent of sexually active people, is considered to be the STD with the greatest risk to fertility. The trouble is that up to 75 per cent of women with this disease and 50 per cent of men have no symptoms. If left untreated, it can lead to PID in women, although for many women once the disease is addressed blocked Fallopian tubes tend to clear up. In my view, although antibiotics will treat the chlamydia, it is still possible that there may be a legacy of inflammation in the body, which can on occasion affect the Fallopian tubes, in turn affecting fertility or increasing the risks of ectopic pregnancy. I see this in terms of Damp and Heat, something which I believe may tend to affect people with a history of STDs (see pages 245–7 for basic advice on Damp and Heat).

Gonorrhea is also associated with a risk to fertility. Up to 25 per cent of women who suffer from this disease will develop PID as a result.

It is thought that herpes, usually signalled by blisters around the genitals, rectum or mouth that take 2–4 weeks to heal, could be linked with elevated natural killer cell activity and implantation failure (see page 219).

For women, the main symptoms of STDs include vaginal discharge, itching and burning in the genital area, pain on urination, pain during intercourse and bleeding between periods. If you do have a history of PID and have any concerns about your fertility, then do talk to your doctor. There are tests (a hysterosalpingogram; see page 250) to check for blockages or scarring. If there is evidence of a problem, then, as with Asherman's, surgery might be an option, or your consultant might advise that IVF is your best bet, depending on your individual case.

For men, there isn't a great deal of research on this subject. It seems that, if left untreated, in the long term chlamydia and gonorrhea can cause inflammation and scarring of the urethra, prostate and epididymus – the connecting tubes from the testicles to the penis. This might cause problems, as will direct contact between sperm and the infection.

ILLNESS AND FERTILITY

So often when I am treating a patient I can trace present problems back to previous illnesses or long-term conditions that then went on to affect their health one way or another for several years. This is why it is so important that when we are unwell or under emotional pressure, we are well nourished, well rested and emotionally supported. It goes a long way to preserving our health and our fertility for the future.

When it comes to a severe illness like cancer, women are understandably often highly concerned for their fertility. Each individual will have her own set of circumstances, so it is vital to talk to your doctor about this concern. Fertility after chemotherapy will tend to be dependent on the intensity of treatment and also on a patient's age. (Good nutrition and acupuncture may go some way to preserving our fertility through chemotherapy.) If the treatment is going to be very intense, there are fertility preservation options including embryo freezing (see page 228), egg freezing and ovarian tissue freezing (see page 34).

YOUR LIFESTYLE

We all feel under increased pressure to pay the mortgage, get a good job, maintain a satisfying relationship and all the other trappings of a successful life. But it won't come as any surprise when I tell you that never having a break and constantly pushing yourself to the limit can cause high levels of stress, leading to adrenal burnout for some and a general frayed feeling for most – that tired-all-the-time sensation. Not getting enough rest is one of the most common factors I notice in women who come to see me. They might fight the commuter crowd in the morning, spend all day in the office and then thrash it out in the gym, which gives a bit of instant relief but goes even further to depleting the energy reserves.

For any woman thinking about or preparing for conception, I always emphasize how helpful a sense of balance in life can be. I am not a very extreme type of person when it comes to diet or exercise or anything else; research shows that fertility is affected both by being overweight and being too thin. I definitely believe in the 'everything in moderation' motto, and this is the case whether we are talking about food, exercise, work or emotions. I have included individual chapters on all of these key fertility factors: diet, exercise and fertility mindfulness. And there are some extra lifestyle factors I want to mention here.

STIMULANTS AND FERTILITY

If you are thinking of getting healthy in order to have a baby or are actively trying to conceive, it won't come as a great surprise that certain stimulants can be less than helpful or even harmful.

Alcohol

The 'everything in moderation' approach is one I tend to advise when it comes to alcohol consumption and fertility. A glass of wine every now and then isn't going to harm your chances of conceiving and has even been shown to be good for our health. It's all about having a good relationship with both food and alcohol so that you don't crave it as a way to relieve stress, for example, but really enjoy it as a healthy part of your balanced life. As with coffee, below, there are times in your cycle when alcohol is best avoided, which I explain in the chapter Your Fertility Diary (see pages 150–8).

Drinking more than an occasional glass of wine and, especially, binge drinking are detrimental to fertility, however. For women, research shows that this type of heavy drinking can stop ovulation and periods, and even moderate drinking can affect regular ovulation.[12] Binge drinking is defined by researchers as drinking six or more units of alcohol in one session for women and eight or more units for men. To give you an idea of what these 'units' really equate to, one 175ml glass of white wine (12 per cent proof) is two units, as is one pint of beer (4 per cent), and a single 25ml measure of spirit like vodka or gin (40 per cent) is one unit. One study found that women who drink fewer than five units of alcohol a week were twice as likely to get pregnant within six months compared to those who drank more.

For men, overconsumption of alcohol can affect sperm quality and count. Alcohol has also been shown to cause cell mutations, plus it has a blocking effect on the absorption of zinc, an important mineral for male fertility.

Binge drinking has become more prevalent in our culture over the past few decades. Whether enjoying a drink out on the town or in the comfort of your own home, the units can easily add up without our even realizing, so it is an important issue to be aware of and address if we want to protect our fertility and be as healthy as possible for pregnancy.

Coffee

Coffee affects people in different ways under different circumstances. When you are chilled out and feeling fantastic on holiday, a cup of coffee may be fine; but it can cause you to feel wired and stressed when you're back at work. Personally I think coffee is better suited to hot countries as it heats the system up and opens the pores, so having a cooling effect, like spicy foods. As with alcohol, if you do enjoy coffee then moderation is essential when you are considering your fertility, and as you'll see in Your Fertility Diary (see page 150), there are certain times of the month when cutting out the caffeine completely can really help. Certain patients benefit from excluding coffee altogether. Increased caffeine consumption affects both male and female fertility. Giving up caffeine may have a seriously beneficial effect on your chances of getting pregnant and of preventing miscarriage.

Smoking and drugs

I'm afraid smoking is a no-no when it comes to fertility (see Changing Habits, Changing Patterns on page 135). Smoking is said to be the cause of 13 per cent of infertility worldwide. Research shows that apart from affecting your overall health, smoking can affect your chances of conceiving and carrying a pregnancy to term.[13] And passive smoking only has a very slightly smaller impact than smoking. Smoking can affect the ovaries and the quality of eggs; it may have a drying effect on the endometrium and can speed up the arrival of the menopause. On average, smokers require twice the number of IVF cycles as non-smokers. Smoking ages you about ten years in terms of fertility. In men, it can affect sperm count and quality, plus quantity of seminal fluid.

And if you use any recreational drugs at all, you need to make sure that you don't get pregnant, as they can cause miscarriage, premature birth and low birth weight as well as inflammation. Recreational drugs appear to have a detrimental effect on what I call our constitutional health (our Jing). This is vital for fertility. Draining this energy in the search for an artificial high can cause fundamental damage and can often affect the emotions too, which are equally vital for fertility health and harmony.

In my clinic, I find it is harder (but not impossible) to improve the fertility of people who took drugs in their youth. Some will get away without too much damage but many won't. Don't forget that if you want a baby later in life the foundations of health need to be in place.

STRESS AND FERTILITY

I believe the emotional stress suffered by women wanting to conceive affects them at the deepest level of their being. It is therefore very important to address the emotional aspects of fertility in order to preserve it and so that emotional distress does not further worsen any physical problems.

Even the word 'stress' sounds tense and negative. We have become so used to hearing how stressed the modern generation is that sometimes we can forget that a little stress is a really good thing, even healthy, as it keeps us motivated and energized. There's nothing like an approaching deadline to suddenly spur on an author, I can tell you! However, with my practitioner's head on, I do also see the negative effects that stress can have on a woman's fertility at first hand. Too much stress plays havoc with our hormones, as well as our weight, sleep, libido, relationships and overall sense of happiness and wellbeing.

The problem with prolonged stress is that it makes our immune systems oversensitive. I liken it to a dimmer switch which never gets properly switched off, constantly hovering on standby. Sustained stress leads to lack of sleep, erratic eating, a feeling of running on empty, all of which contribute to a general state of inflammation. Researchers at Oxford University discovered an association between high levels of stress and reduced chances of a woman conceiving during the fertile days of her cycle.[14] Put simply, too much stress in any one month will reduce your chances of conceiving that month. So managing our stress is a really important part of preserving and helping out our fertility.

CULTIVATING A CALM MIND

What I emphasize to all my patients is that stress manifests very differently in individual women, so when it comes to managing our stress there is no 'one-size-fits-all' instant fix. For lots of women a massage gently encourages them to let go of the need to be in control, which is key for maintaining healthy stress levels. In the chapter Fertility Mindfulness (see page 116) I write about the five different personality types that I identify at my clinic. For each type I explore how stress is likely to manifest, especially in relation to fertility, and some of the ways that I find effective for managing stress in each case.

In recent years mindfulness has entered the mainstream consciousness. Mindfulness is about developing awareness, and I have found that when it comes to fertility the mind plays such an important and very real part. It can be the forgotten piece of the puzzle, so I'm happy to see that gradually this aspect is being considered in greater depth by Western medicine, as I have seen the effects for myself among my patients. I have discussed this subject with many doctors and consultants; because science cannot quite successfully measure it, they find it hard to quantify. Anecdotally, I always think of my mum, who had regular periods all her life, but after my dad died (she was fifty) she never had a period again.

One of the most exciting things I have witnessed through years of treating patients is how belief and expectation can affect outcome in patients. There is an idea that a placebo is inactive, pointless, a sugar pill. I do not believe this to be the case. I think that our belief, our hopes and our minds can have at least some effect on outcome. If we anticipate something is going to be hard, it probably will be, and we create a degree of tension in our body.

I know that my approach to fertility helps bring the body closer to normal function. Many patients report an immediate understanding of their connection to their emotions and how they are impacting on their health. When a person's energies are brought back into alignment, many changes are able to take place, both physically, in terms of fertility and general health, and emotionally. I have witnessed people change many things in their lives as a result; often people find they are able to cope with difficult situations in a calmer, more centred fashion.

CREATING A FERTILITY-FRIENDLY ENVIRONMENT

I spoke to Shideh Pouria, a doctor who specializes in environmental and nutritional medicine (see Resources), about the potential impact factors in our environment can have upon fertility. This is what she said:

> The last century has seen huge changes in our environment, in particular the way we produce food and the types of food we eat. The environmental factors that we are exposed to are vastly different to that of our ancestors, in whom infertility was unusual. There is an increasing awareness that chronic, low-dose exposure to environmental pollutants and toxins may affect fertility and the

developing foetus. These substances are now ubiquitous in our soil, food, air, water, dental materials, prostheses, and products used in our homes and places of work and leisure. Endocrine disruptors are commonplace in our food and immediate environment. It is likely that through repeated exposure they interfere with our reproductive hormones. The effects of environmental oestrogen-like chemicals are well studied in aquatic species and these may potentially impact human reproductive organ function in a similar way. These factors are compounded by nutritional deficiencies that have occurred as a result of modern farming, food manufacturing processes, dietary choices, as well as changes in our bowel microbial flora. Not surprisingly we see a parallel increase in the incidence of allergies and chronic diseases, which in turn may impact conception and successful full-term pregnancies.

My biggest piece of environmental advice when it comes to fertility is to ditch plastic bottles and cellophane, as they can leak oestrogen-mimicking chemicals. Never let a plastic bottle of water heat up in the car before drinking, and whenever possible use filtered water instead, or drink from a glass bottle. I do often wonder about the effect on food that sits around wrapped in plastic packaging. I was in a supermarket once and overheard an elderly woman saying of some plastic-wrapped tomatoes: 'These tomatoes are wonderful – they last two weeks without going off!' You've got to wonder why![15, 16]

Tips on reducing damaging environmental impact in the home

- I recommend natural cleaning products to reduce the chemicals in your immediate environment, as petrochemical compounds disrupt oestrogen.
- Natural, paraben-free beauty products are a good idea too, as are aluminium-free deodorants rather than antiperspirants. Avoid talcum powder when trying to conceive as it can travel up the Fallopian tubes and affect the ovaries.
- Mercury is a heavy metal that can disrupt cell division.
- Dioxins (mainly found in meat and dairy) can disrupt ovarian function.
- Avoid insecticides and pesticides when trying to conceive (ideally avoid at any time).

- Feminine hygiene products are often perfumed and can upset the delicate pH balance of the genital area, so check these carefully and don't use regular soap directly on the genitals.
- Vaginal lubricants are often hostile to sperm – something worth making sure you are aware of!

Even within the past decade men's sperm seems to have changed, with more perfectly healthy men presenting with abnormal or low sperm counts. In my view, some of the things we are exposed to may be having a detrimental effect and causing oxidative stress. We know this can damamge sperm and reduce fertility.

PRESERVING YOUR FERTILITY

It is not always possible for couples to have children earlier in life, and never has preserving our fertility been as relevant as it is now. Women developing their careers often do not feel ready for children until their thirties, or they may not have met the right partner yet. Biologically speaking, some women will be able to conceive well into their forties, but it is vital to take steps to safeguard health and fertility as early as you can.

At my clinic, I have noticed that frequently the problem a patient presents with today can be traced back to something that perhaps might have been prevented or treated more appropriately in the past. For example, an STD that doesn't get diagnosed and results in damaged Fallopian tubes, or a miscarriage that results in retained products and develops into Asherman's, or those months that went past without a period while you thought: 'Great, no periods!'

I believe it is possible for women to put off child rearing until later, but a lot will depend on their genes (their Jing), how well they look after themselves and what life throws at them. Choosing to take steps to preserve your health and look after yourself may pay off in the long run, especially if you delay having a family until later in life. There will always be those who seem to defy all these rules, but I think you will find they are the ones who have the constitution (Jing) of an ox, not mere mortals like the rest of us! Of course, we don't necessarily know which of us will be blessed with a seemingly everlasting supply of eggs or sperm. So it is important not to compare ourselves to others or to celebrities who seem to manage to stay forever young and forever fertile. Take a few simple steps to preserve your health and fertility now – just in case you need it to last a little longer.

In our twenties it is important to avoid STDs, cut down on late nights out and drinking, maintain a healthy body weight and good menstrual cycle awareness. If we can keep our body fit through gentle exercise, we will also be going a long way to helping protect our fertility.

In our thirties, if we are not pregnant then being aware of our gynaecological health is important, as are avoiding STDs, paying attention to how much we might be drinking at home, doing our best to balance work and home life and taking care of our stress levels.

I can't help but think that something called the 'optimism bias' may come into play here. IVF is becoming increasingly successful, but it shouldn't be seen as a safety net: it can't solve all fertility issues for all couples. Don't get me wrong, I am a huge supporter of IVF; but perhaps as a generation we have been slightly oversold it as a fertility 'cure-all'. This might have contributed to a false sense of security and a certain detachment from the reality of how our bodies age, including our fertility. I want to help women reconnect with their fertility.

Of course, you need to feel 100 per cent certain that the time is right for you to have a baby. I completely understand this; I meet lots of women who just aren't ready until a little later than the 'optimum' mid-twenties. In other cases, the women were ready, but their partners were not, and vice versa. The key is to be aware of how your fertility is likely to change throughout your life, and to take steps all along the way to nourish and preserve your fertility for longer.

Most women realize that the optimum fertile period is during our twenties, but just how much is our fertility likely to decline during our thirties and forties? Like most things, much depends on the individual. Again, asking the other female members of your family for their experiences can be really helpful here. Did they have children in their thirties? Did they try for a second baby and struggle with secondary infertility? And if you are able to ask your mother, when did she go through the menopause?

Fertility does begin to noticeably drop from around the age of thirty and then there tends to be a steep decline from thirty-five. By the age of forty, around two in five women trying for a baby will succeed. So if we were just considering biology, trying to start a family before you are thirty-five is a good idea.

However, I know very well that life doesn't always go according to plan or correspond with statistics. And if you only find yourself ready to start a family later, when you're in your thirties, there is much you can do to help increase the likelihood of conceiving. An interesting aside is that you are more likely to conceive non-identical twins in your late thirties, as your body tends to produce more of the follicle-stimulating hormones (FSH) to make you ovulate because there are fewer viable eggs in your ovaries. There is also good news in that while fertility does decline, the vast majority of women still do conceive within three years: 94 per cent of women aged thirty-five and 77 per cent by age thirty-eight.

The decline in fertility for men is more gradual but the number of sperm disorders does increase with age and so it is a factor for men to consider too (see the chapter The Fertile Man, page 42).

AGELESS FERTILITY

In the course of writing this book I talked to several experts on the subject of fertility preservation. For the vast majority of the medical world, fertility preservation equals egg freezing and ageing refers mainly to 'ovarian age', which is determined by a number of tests now available.

I think all of these things are important, and so I will first explain the various tests now available to give an idea of ovarian reserve and rate of ageing. I also consider preservation and ageing to be related very much to the way we live life: what we eat, how we look after our emotions and environmental factors.[17] All of these things make up the foundations for good health and fertility, for better or for worse. So if we take on board some of the basic ideas of living well and in balance, this will go some way towards preserving our fertility. Although the younger we do this the better, it is never too late to make positive changes when it comes to our health.

Ovarian reserve and ovarian ageing

A woman's ovarian reserve is defined by how many follicles or eggs she has left in her ovaries. Ovarian reserve naturally decreases with age, but approximately one-tenth of women experience premature ovarian ageing – that is, their ovarian reserve is found to be lower than expected for their age. Genetic factors are thought to be most significant, but also the extent of oxidative stress on the ovaries caused by environmental and lifestyle factors that are believed to contribute to premature ageing, such as smoking. Recently, the ovarian environment (the conditions in which the follicle/egg maturation processes take place) has been considered to potentially impact on ovarian reserve and ageing. This is interesting, as it supports my own belief that it is not only the egg and the sperm but the reproductive environment and the body as a whole that determine our fertility potential.[18,19]

FSH test

The follicle-stimulating hormone (FSH) test is often used to help evaluate how hard the ovaries will need to work to produce an egg. This can be a helpful indicator of a woman's reproductive capacity. If you know your mum had an early menopause, you might want to think about testing your FSH prior to when you start thinking about wanting to conceive.

AMH test

The anti-Müllerian hormone (AMH) test is used to measure ovarian reserve. In recent years it has become an increasingly popular test to assess a woman's fertility and reproductive age, shown in studies to be an even better predictor of ovarian reserve than the FSH test for women below forty-two years old.[20]

It's important to remember that by your late thirties, an AMH test will naturally show lower levels of ovarian reserve than in your twenties, so don't necessarily be alarmed by the results. While very low AMH has been associated with low chances of conception, there are studies to suggest that pregnancies can still occur and result in live births.[21] And in some instances artificially low results come back, especially when samples are sent off to distant labs. If you do get a bad result, it's a good idea to repeat just to check.

The AMH test is used to indicate the right levels of drugs needed for IVF. If you are put on high doses of drugs as a result of your AMH test, do ask for regular scans to check how many follicles are growing, as some women respond better than expected.

Personally, I find the anti-Müllerian hormone test very emotive: many women will think that a low result means that they will have little or no chance of conceiving, and often this just isn't the case. I use the analogy of glancing into one room of a house and immediately deciding that the whole building needs to be renovated from that one glance. As well as measuring ovarian reserve, we need to look at a patient's overall health, her Fallopian tubes, any other conditions and her medical history. I had a patient who was given her AMH test results over the telephone by a receptionist and in an instant she lost all faith that she would or could have a baby. She was traumatized for years and in the end I believe it became the biggest block to her fertility.

Antral follicle count

This ultrasound scan test is used alongside the AMH test to help determine ovarian reserve. The more follicles are visible, the better it is estimated that you might respond to IVF treatment. I think this is a very worthwhile diagnostic scan and quite an accurate guide to fertility when combined with FSH and AMF tests. It can be used where, previosuly, only surgical diagnostic methods were available.

Bill Smith, head of ultrasound at Clinical Diagnostic Services, talked to me about the advances in 3D transvaginal ultrasound scanning, which has increased our understanding of just how our ovaries change in appearance and activity with age:

Older women have fewer follicles but they tend to be somewhat larger. This might well explain why in women in their forties very often two follicles will reach maturity, hence the increased rate on non-identical twins in older patients. It is also apparent that the stromal tissue within the ovary becomes less glandular and vascular in those patients – perhaps this is why, as we know, fertility status reduces as patients pass forty years of age. Nevertheless, we must not lose sight of the fact that each year many thousands of women naturally conceive in their early or mid-forties, enjoy a normal pregnancy and give birth to a totally healthy baby.

OVARIAN FOLLICLES OVER TIME

FOLLICLES

OVARY

OVER 18 YEARS

UNDER 18 YEARS

20 to 30 YEARS
(IN WOMEN WHO HAVE HAD CHILDREN)

POST-MENOPAUSAL

PERI-MENOPAUSAL

MEDICAL WAYS TO PRESERVE YOUR FERTILITY

Egg banking (oocyte vitrification)

Egg banking is still considered to be the best option in Western medicine for preserving fertility. A woman's eggs are collected at a younger age for potential use later on – usually over the age of thirty-five. It is also offered to cancer patients in certain circumstances (although on occasion the process may be thought to be harmful to treatment). The trouble is that very often women only think about egg banking once it is too late; the cut-off age tends to be thirty-five. Like many things, when it comes to our health we tend to think in the here and now, rather than how to preserve our health for the future. I do think that, in time, the concept of egg banking will become much more mainstream, and young women will be made aware of this option at the right time in their life, rather than when it is a little too late. To date, very few babies have been born from egg freezing.

Generally, two methods are available for egg freezing: slow cooling and vitrification. Recent studies comparing the two methods have demonstrated the superiority of vitrification to slow cooling for egg survival, fertilization and chances of pregnancy.

Ovarian tissue freezing

This is a relatively new approach to preserving a woman's fertility, originally developed to help young women undergoing cancer treatment. The ovary is removed and tissue is then frozen, which can be transplanted back into the woman after remission. It is such a new fertility preservation treatment that we don't yet have the studies to show whether it works, but it is a very interesting development.

The Pill

It is a commonly held misconception that being on the Pill will conserve your egg supply. This is not true. Whether you are on the Pill, pregnant, breastfeeding or not ovulating because you are underweight or overweight, you will still use up your eggs at a constant, predetermined rate each month. If a woman is using the Pill, she might not be using a condom, meaning that the risks for STDs like chlamydia are higher, which could damage fertility. From the perspective of Chinese medicine, although the Pill may preserve Jing, it does so at the expense of the building and moving of Blood, i.e. the natural menstrual cycle, which is vital to fertility.

EGG QUALITY

Egg quality is the Holy Grail in the fertility world. With increasing numbers of couples delaying childbirth, egg quality has never been more relevant. Although we are unable to improve the DNA quality of eggs, which was laid down when we ourselves were embryos, we may be able to affect the mitochondria, which are the cells' power producers. From my own understanding of energy, it makes sense that the quality of the power source for our cells may well be an important factor in improving the integrity of the egg. We do not know the answer to this huge question yet, but in my experience I have noticed that nutrition (including supplements such as CoEnzyme Q10 and L-Carnitine), Chinese herbs and acupuncture can help with Blood flow and influence egg and embryo development and/or implantation for some patients having IVF.

It seems to be slightly easier to improve semen, which is constantly being regenerated, allowing us more influence with acupuncture, healthy lifestyle adjustments and good nutrition.

CoEnzyme Q10

CoEnzyme Q10 is an antioxidant which the body naturally produces less of after the age of thirty. Research is under way to investigate the claims that the supplement CoEnzyme Q10 may improve ovulation and even rejuvenate eggs so that they act like younger eggs – a kind of anti-ageing process for the ovaries. Existing research suggests that the supplement can be linked with higher success rates in IVF, and from a Chinese medicine point of view I consider this supplement good for improving Blood flow, so for patients with scanty Blood flow during their periods I advise taking it post-menstruation.[22]

In men, CoEnzyme Q10 is thought to have a protective action on sperm, improving the count and motility.

DHEA

DHEA is a hormone secreted by the adrenal glands that is converted into fifty other essential hormones, including oestrogens. Between the ages of thirty and fifty, the body's natural production of DHEA declines. DHEA is now used in fertility treatment as it has been shown to overcome decreased ovarian reserve in women by improving or even 'rejuvenating' the ovarian environment. In addition, research shows the hormone may also improve egg quality and embryo numbers, so improving the chances of pregnancy both spontaneously and with IVF (see Resources for where to go for more detailed information).[23, 24] It has also been shown that there is a natural way to improve levels of DHEA: meditation. People over forty-five who regularly meditate have been shown to have up to 47 per cent more DHEA.[25]

Natural ways to improve egg quality and ovarian environment

It may seem an obvious thing to say, but the older you are, the more important it is to take charge of your lifestyle choices. I see many older women who have done just this and in lots of ways are healthier than their younger siblings.

Within the follicular environment, the egg and the follicular fluid together form a functional unit, providing an optimal micro-environment in which the follicle can develop. It is likely that the fluid has both nutritive and protective functions and that environmental factors affecting the follicular fluid will in turn affect the quality of the egg – the lengthy time the egg remains dormant in the ovary provides time and opportunity for environmental factors to take their toll on it.[26] This parallels the belief in Chinese medicine that both the Yin and the Yang that are essential to fertility: Yin being represented by the fluids in the body, the nourishing, protective environment; and Yang being represented by the egg that contains the active fertile potential. So protecting the Yin of the body and ensuring that the follicular fluid is of optimum quality can go some way to improving egg quality in women with poor ovarian reserve (especially when age appears not to be the main factor).

I aim to help women to preserve their Yin and their Blood. I do this through acupuncture, to improve blood flow to the ovaries, but there are also diet and lifestyle ways to keep Yin strong. Yin is the water of the body: it helps to create that nourishing environment for eggs to be produced and later for embryos to grow in the uterus. If you feel you have been overdoing things, if you get hot and bothered or just feel your energy reserves are getting too low, it is an important time of your life to focus on replenishing Yin. Here are some ways you can do this:

- Taking time out for yourself is essential, and rest is especially good in the early days of your period. Don't run around all month long, but try instead to listen to your body's needs.
- Avoid overstimulating foods such as coffee, alcohol, sugar and hot spices.
- Avoid binge drinking.
- Think about environmental factors, as these can be significant; see page 28 for more about this.
- Bird's eggs like chicken, duck or quail are the perfect fertility foods. Other foods that work like a tonic include asparagus, avocado, crab, duck, honey, lemon, mango, milk, nettle, oyster, pea, pear, pomegranate, pork, seaweed, sesame, spelt, spinach, sweet potato, tofu, tomato and watermelon.
- Eat more nuts and seeds, which contain plenty of nourishing essential fats.
- There is some research to suggest that omega-3 essential fatty acids, if consumed within a healthy diet from an early age, may help to strengthen the cell wall and can improve egg quality.[27] These are found particularly in oily fish like mackerel, sardines, trout and salmon.
- If you easily feel cold, then cook warming meals and soups rather than getting by on salads, especially in the winter months.
- Look to support your Jing or essence, which is the foundation of our vitality and so essential for preserving fertility. Balance is the key: between exercise and rest, mental stimulation and relaxation. Foods that boost our essence include almond, bone marrow, chicken, egg, kidney, liver, milk, mussels, nettle, oyster, seaweed, sesame seeds, walnut, caviar (fish eggs), royal jelly, bee pollen and oats.

- Allow yourself to recover fully after major illnesses or life events. Giving yourself time to recover and recuperate from childbirth can be a major factor in preventing secondary infertility (see page 203), and also be kind to yourself and patient with your body after miscarriage (page 201).

A HERBALIST'S VIEW ON OVARIAN PRESERVATION

I spoke to Kate Freemantle, one of the herbalists at my clinic, who has carried out a pilot study investigating ovarian reserve and oriental herbal medicine. This is what she said:

Over the last decade there have been huge advancements in the understanding of women's potential fertility and many new markers to try and estimate ovarian reserve. However, to date, science has yet to clearly unravel the huge complexities of oogenesis and folliculogeneis, i.e. the ability of the ovary to store, activate and grow potential follicles which hold eggs inside.

We still don't have a precise measure on exactly how many eggs a woman has left, what quantity she is releasing for development, how long they take to grow and all that affects the quality of those eggs both positively and negatively.

There is an increasing body of evidence that suggests the microenvironment of the ovary has an important impact on follicular development and that follicles take at least three months to grow to maturity ready for ovulation. This is a long time for the follicles to be 'fed' and supported by the ovaries.

If you take the analogy of a plant seed: for the seed to grow to its optimum, it needs good soil, water, food, sunshine and time. If the environment of the ovary doesn't provide the correct nourishment, then follicles will not develop to their optimum. This is one of the areas where Chinese herbal medicine could potentially help.

MAINTAINING A GOOD WEIGHT

Both overnutrition and undernutrition can have detrimental effects on fertility. It is estimated that 30 to 50 per cent of people of reproductive age are overweight or obese. Increased weight is associated with reduced fertility in both sexes. There is a great deal of focus on women who are obese, but there is also a growing fertility issue with women who are too thin. There is now evidence to suggest that being either extremely over or underweight may have a negative effect on fertility.[28]

Body fat helps convert the male hormone androgen into oestrogen. It's also been shown that having too little body fat can affect the menstrual cycle, and you may stop ovulating even if you are having periods each month. There is also a higher risk of miscarrying in the first trimester of pregnancy.[29]

On the other hand, being overweight can affect your fertility too.[30] You may develop insulin resistance, which can lead to an overproduction of the hormone leptin. This can contribute to irregular ovulation, or again an absence of ovulation altogether. The distribution of fat is also significant. Excess lower body fat around the hips and bottom (pear-shaped) may affect fertility, but to a lesser extent than fat around the middle (apple-shaped).

The simplest way to check if your weight might be impacting on your fertility is to check your BMI (see Resources). The optimum BMI for fertility is considered to be between 20 and 24, so if you are below or above you might want to take steps to lose or gain weight. The good news is that if you eat a healthy diet and take regular exercise, your body will naturally reach a healthy weight, unless you have a pre-existing condition that is affecting your weight, for example a thyroid condition. See In the Fertility Kitchen on page 54 for advice on diet and how to lose weight healthily.

In IVF treatment, studies show that obese women are more likely to yield fewer follicles, fewer eggs are successfully collected and are of poorer quality, and implantation rates are lower, as are rates of pregnancy and live births.[31]

ANTI-AGEING

I asked nutritionist Henrietta Norton (see Resources) for her thoughts on ageing and advice for how to best help slow down the ageing process from a lifestyle point of view. The problems she particularly focuses on are inflammation caused by oxidative stress or free radicals (hence antioxidants being so good for us), toxins, hormonal imbalance and stress that impacts on adrenal function. Of course our bodies age, and much of this is written in our genes, but lifestyle and environment also play a significant part in affecting the rate at which we age, including our fertility.[32] For example, excess stress can produce too much cortisol, which creates an imbalance between the sex hormones oestrogen and progesterone, while diet can either provide our body with plenty of healthy antioxidants which destroy free radicals, or can make the situation worse through overconsumption of foods like refined sugars and saturated fats.

Natural anti-agers

We can slow down the ageing process by eating more foods containing key vitamins and antioxidants:

- Vitamin A – organic liver, eggs and organic dairy
- Vitamin C – bell peppers, papaya, guava, citrus, kiwis, strawberries, broccoli, Brussels sprouts, sweet potatoes
- Vitamin E – wheatgerm, sunflower seeds, hazelnuts, peanuts and almonds
- carotenoids – carrots, squash, oranges and tangerines, green leafy vegetables (especially kale and spinach), tomato products (including puree and tinned tomatoes), apricots, mangoes
- flavanoids – onions, kale, broccoli, apples, tea, red wine, grapes, berries, cherries, green and white tea, apricots, cherries, cocoa and dark chocolate, parsley, thyme, celery
- phenolic compounds – propolis, organic freshly ground coffee, prunes, red wine, vanillin, ginger, chilli
- phyto-oestrogens – soya, pulses, seeds, grain, nuts
- plant sterols – vegetable oils, cereals, nuts, seeds, avocados
- brassicas – Brussels sprouts, cabbage, cauliflower, broccoli, watercress, rocket (better absorbed when lightly cooked rather than raw)
- terpenoids – found in herbs and spices such as mint, sage, coriander, rosemary, ginger

Centre your diet around plant-based foods with as wide an array of colour as possible – include the skin and outer leaves whenever you can if they are organic. By doing this you will optimize your intake of vitamins C and E but also the important phytochemicals, which have potent antioxidant effects. If your fruit and vegetables are not organic, peel the thinnest layer from the top.

Try to reduce your intake of foods that increase free radicals, such as:

- burnt or blackened food
- processed meats – sausages, bacon, ham and other cured meats
- processed foods that contain trans fats

Preventing inflammation

Avoid fats that encourage inflammation such as saturated and trans fats, and increase your consumption of those that reduce the process of inflammation, such as:

- Oily fish, nuts, seeds, avocados and olive oil
- Eat enough lean protein – this is crucial for the maintenance of healthy ovarian function. This includes fish, legumes, grass-fed beef, lamb
- Soya-based foods – miso, tofu, tempeh seem to help prevent some of the processes of ageing
- Green tea – rich in antioxidants needed to repair damaged cells

Acupuncture has also been shown to have an anti-inflammatory effect.[33]

Reducing toxicity in your body

Symptoms of toxic overload include hormonal disruption, fatigue, poor skin or hormonal fluctuations that bring about increased cramps or symptoms of PMS. With toxic overload you become, like so many, the walking 'unwell'.

To optimize detoxification, eat plenty of the foods already listed above and allow your body to take a rest three to four times a year by eating simple foods like soups, congee (rice porridge) and plenty of herbal teas such as fennel, nettle and dandelion for a couple of days.

CHAPTER THREE
THE FERTILE MAN

In my clinic I have a three-month treatment programme for male patients, which is beneficial for simply improving health prior to conceiving, for men who have had a poor semen analysis, or for those whose partner has had repeated miscarriages or unsuccessful IVF treatment. There are some key lifestyle factors men can address which can be extremely helpful when it comes to increasing a couple's chances of getting pregnant. Here are the tips I would give to all men:

- Stop smoking.[34]
- Don't smoke marijuana.
- Take charge of your sexual health: see your GP if you suspect you may have an STD and get checked for any low-grade infections, especially if there is pain when you ejaculate or urinate, or if there is abdominal pain.
- Limit your exposure to any environmental chemicals, and avoid drinking from plastic bottles or heating food in plastic containers.[35]
- If you are overweight, it is a good idea to lose excess weight, as a number of studies have demonstrated a link between excess body weight (especially obesity) and subfertility.
- Exercise is good for sperm, but keep it moderate rather than extreme. Physically active men show better semen results in studies than sedentary men.[36]
- Don't cycle when you are trying to conceive as the pressure cycling places on the perineum may increase the risk of cysts.

- Do pelvic-floor exercises: imagine you are urinating and trying to stop the flow.
- Wear underwear made from natural fibres such as cotton, as it helps the area to keep cool and 'breathe'. I have heard it said that in the 1970s and 1980s when there was a fashion for tight polyester underwear, there was a decrease in men's fertility, but I am not sure if there is any scientific proof of this! Loose cotton underwear is the best option.
- Being exposed to heat is bad for sperm health, so cyclists and chefs, for example, are susceptible to abnormal changes in their sperm. Also be careful of sitting with a laptop directly on your lap. The testicles hang outside of the body so that the sperm can remain cool, so make sure you let it all hang loose when you get the chance. There's nothing wrong with going naked when you are at home. Ditch the saunas, steam rooms and the electric blanket.
- Taking an antioxidant supplement has been shown in studies to improve sperm morphology (health/quality of the sperm).[37, 38]
- Having too much sex is not recommended if you have a low sperm count, although research suggests that abstinence beyond a few days does not improve male fertility, and the majority of couples I see are not having enough sex.
- Sperm quality is improved by regular ejaculation. If you have problems with sperm morphology, aim to have sex three times a week throughout the month, increasing to every other day for a week from day 9 (in a 28-day menstrual cycle).

NUTRITION

- Avoid a high-protein diet, as this may contribute to producing acidic sperm. A healthy diet will help; specific nutrients to include are selenium, zinc, vitamins C and E. Zinc is found in oysters, pumpkin seeds, rye, oats, almonds and peas. Selenium is present in tuna, sesame seeds, shellfish, avocados and wholegrains.
- Other good foods to include are oily fish, peppers, broccoli, cauliflower, cabbage, spinach, chicken and fish.
- Ginseng supplements improve the blood flow to the penis and may improve sexual function in some patients.

- Avoid consuming too much alcohol: it can be a cause of low sperm count and impaired sperm motility.
- Avoid eating too many soya products, as overconsumption has been shown to affect sperm quality.

EATING THE RIGHT KIND OF FAT

A study by Harvard Medical School discovered that men with a diet high in saturated fats produced significantly less sperm (and weaker quality sperm) than men who ate a healthy, balanced diet.[39]

Male patients attending a fertility clinic were questioned about their diet and fat intake. The results showed that junk food not only carries health risks like heart disease, obesity and cholesterol, but it can also damage sperm count and sperm quality. Men who regularly ate junk food had a 43 per cent lower sperm count and a 38 per cent lower sperm concentration (the number of sperm per unit volume of semen) compared to men who ate healthily.

Researchers also discovered that a diet rich in omega-3 fatty acids is best for boosting sperm quality.[40] Foods rich in omega-3 fatty acids include oily fish (such as sardines, mackerel and salmon) and flax seeds.

FACTORS IN MALE SUBFERTILITY

Male subfertility (lower quality or quantity of sperm) may be a factor for at least half of all couples experiencing infertility, and it is a growing problem throughout the world. It appears as though male fertility may be more susceptible to environmental factors, and yet medicine tends to focus much more on female infertility when it comes to treatment and intervention.

Here are some of the factors that can play a role in male subfertility.

- age
- undescended testicles

- varicocele (enlargement of veins in the scrotum)
- lifestyle and environment
- too much Heat
- testicular cancer (and other cancers treated prior to conceiving)
- vasectomy
- STDs

Semen analysis

The causes of male infertility are divided into two categories: physical abnormalities of the male reproductive tract, and abnormalities of the sperm. In most cases, the cause will be unknown, but semen analysis is still very helpful to determine a man's fertility potential. The information provided by a semen analysis test includes:

- sperm quality (motility and morphology) and count
- male reproductive hormone balance
- condition of reproductive tract
- infections of the reproductive glands, such as the prostate gland
- congenital abnormalities

Understanding your semen results

The World Health Organization has suggested that there are no 'normal' values for semen analysis, because men with results that lie outside the considered 'normal' range may actually be able to father a child. But results can suggest whether men will find it more difficult to conceive and may signpost the best treatments.

Sperm DNA fragmentation test

Sperm also suffer negative effects of ageing and seemingly healthy-looking sperm from a semen analysis can still contain high levels of DNA fragmentation, something which can cause male infertility.[41] Increased sperm DNA fragmentation is associated with infection, diet, drug use, smoking, environmental toxins, age, heat exposure to testicles, varicocele and other medical conditions. Some causes cannot be treated, but if it is thought to be lifestyle-related then changes to lifestyle can help, including a diet rich in antioxidants (see page 40) designed to reduce oxidative stress.

According to consultant gynaecologist James Nicopoullos, we now know that even men with perfectly normal sperm counts can have a high level of DNA damage in their sperm, which can affect their chances of getting their partners pregnant naturally. However, the use of techniques such as ICSI and more recently IMSI (see page 230 for more details) to inject sperm directly into eggs seems to overcome such damage. Recently men with varicocele have been shown to have an increase in levels of DNA damage; in this scenario varicocele removal may also be prudent.

MALE FERTILITY PRESERVATION: SPERM FREEZING

There are a number of reasons why it might be advisable to consider freezing semen:

- cancer diagnosis
- medication
- fertility-threatening surgery
- ejaculation dysfunction
- PESA or TESE treatment (in men with azoospermia)
- prior to vasectomy

The effects of paternal age on fertility are clearly minimal compared to those of the age of the female partner. Testicular volume and possible function only decrease towards the eighth decade of life. There may be a small increase in the proportion of genetically abnormal sperm with increasing age, but in a far more limited way than the steady depletion of egg reserve and egg quality with age.

So, beyond sperm banking prior to any possible chemotherapy or radiotherapy in a man of reproductive age, the advice to men for preserving fertility predominantly revolves around lifestyle. It is clear that smoking negatively affects sperm concentration, motility (movement) and the proportion of normal sperm, as well as impacting negatively on the genetics of sperm. Recent studies have suggested that male BMI may also correlate with the outcome of fertility treatment, with a reduction in live births from IVF with increasing BMI and a poorer embryo development rate.[42]

Acupuncture

Acupuncture is beneficial in raising general health and vitality levels in men. Extensive research has also shown acupuncture to be effective in improving sperm count, motility and morphology.[43] After an initial course of acupuncture, I often recommend that men receive more treatments around the time of their partner's ovulation.

PART TWO
GETTING HEALTHY FOR PREGNANCY

This is the best thing you can do for your children – more important than money, education, extra tuition or a fancy bedroom. Good health is a gift and it is the best gift you can pass on to the next generation.

SEASONS AND CYCLES

When speaking of one day the morning is governed by spring, the afternoon by summer, evening by fall and night by winter. The spring energy gives birth, the summer produces maturity, the fall is the time for gathering in, and the winter is a time for storage.

Nei Ching, *The Yellow Emperor's Classic of Internal Medicine*

I am very aware of the influence the seasons can have on our health. I see how my patients' energy changes throughout the year. As developed as human beings have become, we are still part of nature and what happens to our environment happens to us. Cycles are a part of the rhythm of life; to stay in good health, we do well to connect with the cycles of the year and those within our bodies.

Summer is the most expansive time of year: it is when we have the most available energy and the days are longest. It is the time of year for going out and mingling with our fellow human beings. The summer is when we store up joy for the rest of the year. I always say to patients who have been trying to conceive for a long time: 'Let go, enjoy yourself and try to engage in life as much as possible.' In summer we don't have to be so strict with ourselves. It's good to rediscover the laid-back you and just go with the flow a bit more. It is about 'doing things' rather than 'having things to do'. If you eat well most of the time, there is no harm in letting things slip a little – part of a balanced life is losing balance occasionally. It's fine to burn the candle a little longer in the summer; it will do your Heart some good and bring a little joy back into your life.

In late summer things begin to get back to normal. It feels like 'back to school' time. It's about getting organized again and beginning to knuckle down. It's a good time to bring your attention back to having a baby and make a gentle plan about going forward, as this is the traditional time of year for starting new projects. If you are trying to conceive, set yourself a few goals and a time scale. The fertility journey can become very linear, punctuated only by the monthly arrival of your period. Try to make a three-month plan, say, to get healthy, and then review progress. If you have been trying for a while, make a plan to seek advice from a professional. Start to clean up your diet a bit: bring your focus back to nourishing foods and reduce the amount of sugar and dairy in your diet. If you have had the odd few drinks over the summer, it's time to get back on track and be a bit healthier again.

Autumn and winter are really when energy begins to move inwards and we have less of it. It's a time of year for conserving our energy. Many animals hibernate in the winter and grow lovely warm coats to keep themselves warm. My rule in the winter is 'nothing good happens after midnight' – in the summer I let this rule slip occasionally. So keep warm, have early nights, go out less and eat more hot cooked foods that will warm you to your centre. Nurture yourself. Slow-cooked foods are good as they release their heat slowly and warm your body to its core. Avoid a radical diet or detox in the New Year – it is a ridiculous time to limit your calorie intake and to dramatically change your eating habits. By all means avoid alcohol, sugar and processed foods and live a bit more healthily, but please don't start eating raw food in the middle of winter as it is completely counterintuitive and will only slow your system down and make your core colder, which is not good for fertility.

In spring you will be coming alive again. As everything buds and sprouts around us in nature, so we do too. This is the time of year when there is the most opportunity for growth and the most energetic potential. Everything around us is reawakening. Now you can afford to make your diet a little lighter, but don't skip meals and don't fast. Maintaining balanced blood-sugar levels is very important for your fertility, which means eating regularly and not skipping meals. You can add some sprouting seeds to your diet and more salads as well. But do keep some cooked foods in your diet to maintain a balance.

When making a fertility plan with a patient, I do often consider the time of year. For example, if a patient is considering doing IVF, and time is on her side age-wise, it might be worth considering the timing of it in terms of where we are in the year. If it's January, I may well advise her to dedicate a few more months to preparation as we move into the spring, as there will be more energy available to her, plus lighter days. In spring and summer it does feel as though we have more hours in the day. Equally, if it's September and we are about to head into autumn and winter, I might be tempted to suggest that she does her IVF before the days get shorter and while she is feeling healthy and well after the summer. There is not much scientific evidence to support this, but anecdotally patients report that they have more success in the springtime. Certainly I usually see a little flurry of increased pregnancy rates in spring and summer, so it might be a factor to bear in mind.

To patients trying to conceive naturally, I might say let's start this new plan in September, giving them the summer to relax and gently think about the changes they are going to make and then begin in earnest after that. It will be slightly different for everyone, and will also depend on their workload and job and many other things. But it is often a gentle consideration when putting together a fertility plan.

Whatever the time of year, it is important to adjust our activities according to how we feel. Listen to your body: we will all feel better at some times than at others; some of us thrive in the winter, for example. Knowing yourself and making a connection with your environment is an important part of preserving your health and fertility. If you know you are less energetic in winter, don't burn the candle at both ends and don't overdo it. I know myself how the year can pan out – being a medical practitioner, I am governed the entire year by appointments in my diary. So my rule to myself is that (outside of diary bookings), nothing much gets put in the diary as a fixed plan in the summer months. It is my time to be free and spontaneous as much as I possibly can. In terms of work commitments, around June I start postponing new projects until September to give me the time I need to prepare and start to make some space in my life. I am a big believer that if we don't actually make the space for new things, then it is very hard for us to embrace anything new at any time, as there is literally no room in our life.

It's important to have these disciplines, however small they are, to make sure that the year has an ebb and flow – just like our life and our own menstrual cycles.

CHAPTER FOUR
IN THE FERTILITY KITCHEN

Diet and fertility are two of the major health and wellbeing issues for modern women. On the whole we are all much more aware these days just how important our diet is; television programmes, magazine articles and shelves of books are available on how to eat more healthily. Clearly this is a positive trend, as a good diet provides the building blocks for good health. More than that, particular foods can even be used to address some conditions and give people a great tool to enrich their lives and their health. If you look after your diet, you will certainly be going a long way to taking care of your fertility.

Food and fertility are intimately linked. Our diet affects our hormones and our overall health. We can choose foods that support the different phases of the menstrual cycle, we can nourish our energy, warm ourselves when our bodies feel Cold or cool them in times of Heat. Food is one of nature's incredible helping hands; I could write whole books on the benefits of tea or chicken soup. I am never more content than when creating in the kitchen. Food is life, after all. It helps us to do something loving for ourselves and those we care for. Part of being or becoming fertile is the ability to receive nourishment for ourselves on both a digestive and emotional level. As we learn to do this for ourselves, so we will be better able to do so for another human being.

The fertility cycle is connected with the cycles of nature, and also the cycles of our life, from puberty through to post-menopause. In the modern world we often think of everything as linear: where are we going and how are we going to get there. But of course everything in nature, including our bodies, is cyclical, from the rising and setting of the sun to our menstrual cycles to the seasons. There are four phases to each menstrual cycle, just as there are four seasons. So it is good to eat certain foods and drink particular teas during these four phases, for example Blood-nourishing foods such as beetroot and aubergine after menstruation in the follicular phase.

Nature, in her turn, tends to provide many of the right foods for us through the seasons. During the winter, we need the warmth of sweet root vegetables, while in the summer it really does pay to be as cool as a cucumber. There is a growing trend to associate raw foods and juices with cleansing the body or losing weight, especially in January after the excesses of the holidays. The trouble is that we are loading our systems with cold foods that are much more suited to the height of summer at a time when we need warmth and lots of nourishment to keep our immune and digestive systems firing on all cylinders. In fact, eating cold, raw foods in cold weather actually weakens the digestive system.

DITCH THE FAD DIETS

The trend towards high-protein or low-fat diet regimes might be making women lean, but fertility health (and happiness) is suffering. Popular diets usually try to be one-size-fits-all, rather than bespoke and aimed at the individual. Often they will limit certain food groups which should be part of a healthy balanced diet. Certain fats, like the omega-3s found in oily fish and avocados, are essential both for health and fertility. Plus many low-fat foods contain sugar or artificial sweeteners instead of fat to give them taste, which, ironically, have been shown to cause weight gain and are not helpful for fertility either. One example: whole milk has been shown to be far more beneficial to fertility than skimmed.[44] Wholegrain 'slow' carbohydrates that are digested slowly have been shown to be beneficial, while 'fast' sugars that upset our blood sugar balance are shown to be upsetting for our hormone balance too, so can affect ovulation. Too much animal protein is unhealthy, while protein and iron from plant-based sources is very good for us.

The other important thing to remember is that very few, if any, weight-loss diets are written with conception in mind. The desired outcome is a red-carpet, beach-ready body. The fertile body can be toned, but it also has a softness and is receptive. Some very popular diets feature gallons of water and lots of raw food. This might suit some people, but for others all that raw food will slow down the metabolism and too much water, especially around meal times, floods the digestion and stops vital digestive enzymes working, so that we don't absorb all the nutrients in our food. We tend to have forgotten along the way that much of our hydration can come from food itself, rather than ice-cold water. Soups, for example, are wonderful for hydrating and nourishing at the same time.

Fad diets rarely take into consideration climate or seasons, so we might end up drinking vegetable juices all day long in the middle of winter while there is snow on the ground, when a vegetable stew would be so much more nourishing. As I will show you in the section Your Fertility Diary, eating slightly different foods and amounts of food during the four phases of the cycle can be incredibly beneficial to body and mind. For example, we need to fire up our digestive furnaces around ovulation and in the second half of the cycle, while it's a good idea to eat lighter, simpler foods after our periods.

HEALTHY WEIGHT LOSS

While I'm not a diet expert, helping women (and a few men) to lose weight healthily is definitely part of what I do as a specialist in women's health and fertility. I don't promise any quick-fix solutions, but I do offer core principles plus a few weight-loss wonder foods that lead to gentle weight loss that lasts, boosting your fertility, energy and general wellness levels.

It is very important to lose weight slowly, because rapid weight loss damages the digestion and so makes it much harder in the long run to keep the weight off. When you try to lose weight with a crash diet, the body goes into survival mode and will think it is starving. Not only does your system then hold on to every calorie it can, slowing down your metabolism, but it may also have a negative effect on fertility.

Tips for healthy weight loss
- Try not to worry too much about calories; think about the quality of the foods you eat instead. Go for fresh, unadulterated and natural foods wherever possible and get the body moving.
- Don't cut out fat. Essential fats will help you lose weight, especially those found in oily fish, avocado, olive oil, coconut oil and sesame.
- Eat regularly and don't skip meals.

RESOLVE DAMP TO LIGHTEN UP

For most people, eating a diet that resolves any Damp in the body is perfect if you need to lose weight. This means including plenty of the following foods:

- aduki beans
- alfalfa
- asparagus
- barley
- basil
- broad beans
- buckwheat
- caraway
- cardamom
- celery
- clams
- cloves
- coriander
- corn
- duck

- fenugreek
- garlic
- grapes
- green tea
- horseradish
- jasmine tea
- kidney beans
- lemon
- lettuce
- mackerel
- mung beans
- mushrooms
- mustard leaf
- onions
- oregano

- parsley
- peas
- pumpkin
- quail
- radishes
- rice
- rye
- sardines
- seaweed
- squash
- turnips
- watercress
- umeboshi plums

- Don't flood the digestion with too much water during mealtimes, but sip room temperature water or warm herbal teas throughout the day.
- Raw food tends to constrict the digestion. Rather than choosing salads for every meal, go for soups instead.
- Add a little sweetness with a small amount of honey, and avoid refined sugars.[45]
- Eat more in the morning and less in the evening to fire up your digestion first thing and let it rest and recover overnight.
- Don't think of vegetables and grains only as side dishes. There are so many vegetarian recipes even in this book that make a great meal, using ingredients like aubergines, beans, quinoa and squash.

- Remember that if you add some light exercise to your day then you'll be helping to fire up your Qi and your digestion. Increase the amount you exercise gradually as you get stronger and healthier.
- Eat as rich a variety of foods as possible. Many food intolerances arise because we eat such a restricted diet, for example eating mostly wheat when there are so many grains to choose from, like barley, bulgur, rye, oats and spelt.
- Don't aim for perfection: aim for good enough and don't compare yourself to others. It is important to shift excess weight, but acceptance of who you are and your body type is vital too.
- Look for any emotional issues behind your eating habits. I've included some websites and books on the emotions of eating at the back of the book (see Resources). The section on Fertility Mindfulness will also help you to be more aware of your emotions and how they may affect your lifestyle.[46]

DIGESTION IS EVERYTHING

While debates and discoveries about what constitutes the healthiest diet go on, something is often missing from all the discussion, and that's the importance of digestion. Because the benefits of even the most impeccable diet can be seriously diluted by a faulty digestive system.

It is important to take into account the entire state of the abdominal cavity, as well as the ovaries and uterus. The role of the bowel is very important: a bowel that functions below par can impact the general flow of the cycle. In accordance with Chinese medicine, I always view the body as a whole and not as separate subsections such as reproduction and digestion, as if one has no bearing on the other, and I would encourage you to do the same.

Having a good appetite is a sign of good digestive health. This does not mean that you should be constantly hungry, only that you are appropriately hungry. I have noticed that these days many women seem to place value on a lack of appetite, as it makes them feel in control of their eating, but this is not a good sign in terms of digestion. It is really important to cultivate a healthy approach to eating and to be good to yourself, because our thought process and digestion are connected; the stomach is even described as the body's second brain by scientists. And in my field, it is thought that obsessing or feeling negative about food can affect our ability to absorb nourishment from what we eat.

LISTENING TO YOUR BODY

Recently a woman came to my clinic to be treated for fertility problems. As we talked, I discovered she had been taking twenty-eight different vitamins and supplements every day. I had already taken her medical history and established her digestion was functioning below par. She suffered from loose stools, bloating and a tendency to ruminate and worry a great deal. A tendency to overthink is often a sign that the digestion is poor; in the same way that the person is unable to assimilate and absorb thoughts and ideas, they are also unable to assimilate and absorb nutrients from the food they eat. The patient's tongue was swollen with teeth marks down each side, another indication that her digestion was weak. Taking such high levels of vitamins and minerals is really a waste of time and money and can even cause more damage than good. It is, if you like, a case of being 'overly nutritious': the levels are hard for the body to digest, putting further strain on the system, further weakening the digestion.

Supplements can be extremely helpful in the right circumstances (see page 100). But sometimes we need to work on the digestion first. As a general rule, I am of the belief that the majority of our nutrition needs to come from food; if our diet is healthy and varied and our digestion is strong then we get everything we need. With this in mind, one of the first things I do with a new patient is not only to ask them what they eat, but also how, when and why they eat.

YOU ARE WHAT, HOW, WHEN AND WHY YOU EAT

We have known for some time that 'we are what we eat', but have you ever considered the who, when, how and why of what we eat? Most of us are pretty up to speed on what constitutes a healthy diet. Personally, I believe there are very few real foods that are inherently 'bad'. Sugar and dairy get a very bad press, for example, but small amounts are fine for most people; it's really a question of quantity and quality. Of course, consuming large amounts of refined sugars is unhealthy, but a small amount of natural sugars in the diet is actually very good for our digestion. The same with milk – a small amount in its most natural state does have health benefits.

The 'who' of food

Another consideration is *who* is eating the food, for 'one man's meat is another man's poison'. We are all different and we can all tolerate different foods at different times. For some, a spicy curry is a treat, while others can't stand the heat. Dairy for some is too 'Dampening' – it makes their bodies form excess mucus and can aggravate any Damp-type condition they may have, for example asthma, cystitis, skin conditions such as eczema; it may even slow down ovulation. So the trick is to not compare yourself with other people and to be aware that your nutritional needs may change with your changing body and the changing seasons.

The 'when' of food

The stomach likes to be regularly fed; it does not like erratic eating patterns. So 'when' you eat can have a big bearing on how well your body absorbs what you eat. Eating every three to four hours is ideal and will keep your blood sugars balanced. Very often I have patients explain to me what a healthy diet they have, and yet after further scrutiny it turns out that for a large period of time during the day they are literally starving. Remember that regular mealtimes are best for your stomach and blood sugars. I do think it's fine to have a couple of days a week when you reduce your intake of food (as long as you are not underweight), but you should still eat regularly, just smaller amounts.

The 'how' of food

How we eat, in terms of our environment, is also a consideration. If you always eat breakfast on the go or at your desk while doing your work, this will have an impact on your digestion. I think it's important to make space for food and to make it a priority, like the French, who steadfastly stop for lunch to take a break from their work and digest their food. It's important and your digestion will thank you for it.

Don't:
- eat while working
- eat while travelling, such as when standing on a bus or train
- eat while doing business

- eat while worrying
- eat while arguing
- obsess about food
- flood the digestion with too much liquid

Do:
- chew your food well: remember 'the stomach has no teeth'
- make proper times to eat
- talk about joyful things
- engage in food and the process of eating: be mindful
- think about what you are eating and how it got to your table

The 'why' of food

So many people eat for the wrong reasons, or don't eat much at all. For many, food has become an obsession – a way of feeling they have some control over themselves, when perhaps they don't. Denying yourself nourishment is a deep imbalance and one that might need addressing professionally. Equally, overeating is a huge problem in society and behind every overweight person is an emotional issue crying out to be heard (see Resources for contact details of Overeaters Anonymous).

Our ability to nourish ourselves or deny ourselves nourishment goes to the very heart of who we are and our relationship with ourselves. Our ability to receive nourishment on every level is tied up with our feelings of self-worth. For many women (and men) this can become a lifelong battle.

Think about why you do or don't eat and look for the emotional impulse behind what drives that – you may find it has little to do with food and more to do with mind and Heart.

WEAK DIGESTION

If you suffer from any of the following signs of weak digestion, you should incorporate the tips below, in addition to the Tips for Eating Well on page 62, to give your digestive fire a helping hand:

- loose stools
- constipation

- excess wind
- bloating
- digestive cramps

How to strengthen your digestion

Try the food combining approach. This was developed in the 1920s by Dr Howard Hay and it can help your body digest foods more easily. Think of foods as three groups: proteins, carbohydrates and neutral foods. Proteins and carbohydrates should not be eaten together while neutral foods can be eaten with either proteins or carbohydrates.

Proteins include: meat, fish, shellfish, dairy, eggs, tofu and any soya foods.

Carbohydrates include: grains, potatoes, sweet potatoes, fruits and sugars (including honey and maple syrup).

Neutral foods include: vegetables, herbs, spices, mushrooms, yoghurt, nuts, seeds, oils and fats.

- Take extra care not to work and eat at the same time.
- Include foods that soothe and support the digestion, like carrots, squash and sweet potato.
- Steer clear of too many raw foods, as your digestion isn't strong enough to handle these.
- Avoid overstimulating foods and drinks, like hot spices, caffeine and alcohol.
- Take a probiotic supplement to help your gut flora.

TIPS FOR EATING WELL

If you eat as many natural and seasonal foods as possible, you will be going a long way towards maintaining a healthy, fertility-friendly diet. Try not to worry too much about what you eat; it is important that you feel good about what you digest. So as long as your diet is generally healthy, don't beat yourself up about the occasional indulgence. Don't obsess about food or be too controlling about what you consume.

I would say that it is important to try to avoid processed foods or ready meals as much as possible. Here are some other tips to follow:

- Enjoy rich foods like meat or dairy, but in moderation.
- Include plenty of vegetables, beans and legumes, oily fish and grains.
- Steer clear of eating too much sugar, especially in its refined state, as it interferes with the body's natural balance and has an ageing effect.
- Avoid stimulants like alcohol and coffee, especially in the first half of your cycle. The odd one is fine for most people – 'on high days and holidays' as my mum says.
- Slow down and chew your food: aim for 20 mouthfuls in 20 minutes.
- Eat regularly and do not skip meals.
- Do not flood the digestion: don't drink lots of fluids with your meal. Keep liquids, especially cold drinks, to a minimum; instead take most of your liquids away from mealtimes.
- Eat mostly cooked foods and avoid eating cold food straight out of the fridge. The digestion likes food that is warm and cooked, particularly in cold and damp climates like the UK.
- 'Eat light and live long': do not overeat and remember to stop when you are about two-thirds full (your brain takes a little while to catch up and know that you are actually full).
- Do not read while eating: remember that thinking and digesting are a similar function and the body sometimes struggles to achieve both at once.
- At work, eat your food away from your desk and try to walk around the block or at least get some fresh air after eating.
- Do not argue or discuss contentious issues while you eat: it knots up the stomach and slows down digestion.

THE FERTILITY STORE CUPBOARD

Below I have listed foods and recipes for each of the four phases of your cycle. Included are the key fertility foods that nutritionists will recommend for a balance of good protein, essential fats, complex carbohydrates, fibre, antioxidants, vitamins and minerals. I am not a nutritional therapist, but as part of my training I studied Chinese food dynamics, which teaches you the energetic qualities of food. I consider food to be part of medicine. When I myself am unwell, before turning to stronger medicine I will first adapt my diet and then reach for the acupuncture needles. In our house, food is used medicinally as part of everyday life: a bit of ginger here; a calming tea there; a reduction in dairy and sugar in the autumn. I constantly make minor or major adjustments; it's an alchemy of sorts. I think much can be achieved by giving the body the correct conditions to 'be well', and food is always my starting point.

Here are my general recommendations for a fertility-friendly diet:

- Eat plenty of fresh fruit and vegetables for vitamins, minerals, fibre and antioxidants (especially all the brightly coloured fruit and veg). Variety is key here – don't stick to just one favourite fruit or veg.
- Nuts, seeds, avocados and oily fish are good sources of essential fatty acids, which help to balance hormones and nourish all of the cells in our body.
- Lentils, beans and pulses help with hormone regulation, plus they are good sources of fibre too.
- Tofu and tempeh are good for balancing sex hormones; they are also thought to be helpful for conditions including fibroids (see page 197) and endometriosis (see page 191).
- Grains help to balance blood sugar and give us sustained energy throughout the day; they are also good for balancing moods and provide another healthy source of fibre.
- Small amounts of meat are a good source of protein and iron.
- Eggs are an excellent source of protein and are quick and easy to prepare.

Emotions, particularly stress, anxiety and worry, can hinder the absorption of nutrients, like my patient who was taking masses of supplements but was still undernourished. I really encourage you to read the chapter on Fertility Mindfulness, as food is so connected with our emotions. Once we have developed a healthy relationship with food, our overall health and vitality seems to improve in leaps and bounds.

EATING THROUGH YOUR CYCLE

Phase 1: During your period

During this phase you should look to include foods that encourage movement of Blood out of the body, to promote the complete discharge of the old endometrial lining. Aubergines are a good example. Avoid sour foods, which are astringent and inhibit the flow of Blood, like yoghurt, pickles, oranges and grapefruit.

Blood-moving foods:

- aubergines
- brown sugar
- butter
- chestnuts
- eggs
- chilli
- chives
- crab
- kohlrabi
- leeks
- mustard leaf
- onions
- peaches
- radishes
- saffron
- spring onions
- sticky rice
- turmeric
- vinegar

Blood-nourishing foods (very good for just after your period ends)

- aduki beans
- apricots
- beef
- beetroot
- bone marrow
- cherries
- eggs
- dandelion
- dates
- figs
- grapes
- kale
- kelp
- kidney beans
- leafy greens
- liver
- mussels
- nettle
- octopus
- oysters
- parsley
- sardines
- seaweed
- spinach
- squid
- sweet rice
- tea: rose or nettle
- tempeh
- watercress

Recipes

STEAK WITH QUICK ROAST BEETROOT AND MUSTARDY GREENS

This is excellent for lunch or an early dinner, but don't eat meat too soon before bedtime. Use a mixture of whatever warming mustardy greens you can get: dandelion, mustard leaf, rocket and watercress all work well. They are good for your digestion as they are warming, but they also relieve Stagnation. The orange peel, coriander and caraway will help too.

Serves 2
2 150g rib-eye steaks
few sprigs of thyme
1 orange
1 tbsp Dijon mustard
extra-virgin olive oil
6 vacuum-packed beetroots in natural juice
1 tsp coriander seeds
1 tsp caraway seeds
1 tbsp red wine vinegar
2 big handfuls of mustardy greens
sea salt and freshly ground black pepper

1. Preheat your oven to 180°C/350°F/gas mark 4. Quickly marinade your steaks – even marinating for just 5 minutes will give you some extra flavour. Put the steaks in an ovenproof dish. Pull the thyme leaves off the stalks and throw them over the steaks, then use a fine grater to grate the orange zest onto the steaks and dollop half the mustard on top of each one. Add a glug of olive oil and then use your hands to rub all the flavours into the steaks.

2. Cut the beetroot into quarters and put into a roasting tray. Crush the coriander and caraway seeds in a pestle and mortar and tip onto the beetroot. Pour over the vinegar and a glug of oil, season with salt and pepper and mix well. Roast in the oven for 25 minutes until the beetroot is crisping round the edges.

3. When the beetroot is nearly ready, heat a griddle pan until smoking hot, season the steaks with salt and pepper and griddle for 3 to 4 minutes on each side for medium-rare (cook for another minute or so on each side if

you like them well done). Allow the steaks to rest for a minute while you dress the mustardy greens in the juice of half of the orange, some olive oil and a pinch of salt and pepper.

4. Serve the steaks next to a pile of beetroot and a sprightly handful of mustardy greens.

Aubergine three ways

Aubergines are wonderful for moving the Blood, so much so that I suggest not eating them in early pregnancy. If you think about the shape and colour of an aubergine, it actually looks a bit like a uterus, so it does not take a lot of imagination to see that it may have the ability to stimulate Blood in the uterus. This makes it potentially very helpful for women who suffer from painful periods or periods that tend to stop and start.

SPICED AUBERGINE RATATOUILLE

Ginger is an anti-inflammatory, while the fenugreek helps with uterine contractions and movement of Blood.

> **Serves 4**
> *groundnut oil*
> *2 large aubergines, diced*
> *2 onions, finely sliced*
> *thumb-sized piece of ginger, finely chopped*
> *1 clove of garlic, cut into slithers*
> *1 tsp ground cumin*
> *1 tsp ground coriander*
> *1 tsp turmeric*
> *2 tsp fenugreek seeds*
> *400g chopped tomatoes*
> *1 tbsp each of chopped coriander and mint*
> *Greek yoghurt to serve*

1. Sauté the aubergine in the groundnut oil until lightly browned and drain on kitchen paper. Cook the onions in a tablespoon of groundnut oil until very soft and translucent. Add the ginger, garlic and spices and stir for a minute, then add the tomatoes and a splash of water and cook for

30 minutes until the sauce is reduced. Add the aubergine and cook for 15 minutes on a low heat.

2. Serve with brown basmati rice, sprinkle with coriander and mint and add some yoghurt on the side.

BABAGANOUSH WITH HOMEMADE PITTA-BREAD CHIPS

A perfect snack for this phase in your cycle. Pack into little tubs to combat energy lows, or eat as a light lunch with some zingy lemon-dressed salad. A little pomegranate molasses drizzled over the top of your finished dip adds interest, but is by no means a necessity.

Enough for 10 snack-sized portions
3 large aubergines
2 cloves of garlic, peeled and finely chopped
3 tbsp tahini
juice of 1 lemon
pinch of toasted cumin seeds
4 tbsp extra-virgin olive oil
sea salt and freshly ground black pepper
4 round pitta breads
few sprigs of fresh mint
olive oil

1. Prick the skins of the aubergines with a fork. Place them over a gas flame or a barbecue or under a hot grill and char for 5 to 10 minutes, turning often with tongs until they are evenly charred and the flesh is soft all the way through. Allow to cool a little before cutting in half and scraping out the flesh. Discard the skins and place the flesh in a bowl with the tahini, lemon, cumin and extra-virgin olive oil and mix well.

2. Cut the pittas into eight pieces and place on a baking tray with a drizzle of olive oil and some salt and pepper. Bake in the preheated oven for 10 minutes until crisp and golden on the corners.

3. Serve the babaganoush sprinkled with the chopped mint and the warm pitta chips.

BAKED AUBERGINE TAPENADE

Serves 4

1 large aubergine
2 smallish bell peppers – red, yellow, green or orange
1 small onion
3 large garlic cloves
extra-virgin olive oil
sea salt
thyme, rosemary and basil, fresh or dried – ½ tsp of each if dried; a
   few sprigs or leaves of each if fresh
1 lemon (zest and juice)
dried chilli flakes or cayenne pepper (optional)

1. Preheat the oven to 220°C/425°F/gas mark 7. Rinse the aubergine and cut into 2-inch pieces. Core and seed the peppers and cut them into quarters. Peel and slice the onion into quarters and then into 2-inch pieces. Peel the garlic cloves. On a large baking tray arrange all the vegetables, coating them with olive oil and sea salt and adding the herbs if dried – if fresh, just add the thyme and rosemary. Loosen the onion slices, add the dried chilli flakes or cayenne pepper if using and add a little of the zest of the lemon. Bake in the oven for 15–20 minutes. Start checking after about 13 minutes: the aubergine slices should be soft in the middle when done, and the peppers, onions and garlic slightly browned, but not charred. Remove from the oven and allow to cool.

2. When cooled, chop all the bigger pieces into bite-sized cubes and place in a serving bowl. If you're using fresh basil, tear up the leaves and add to the tapenade. Mix together, taste and season. Squeeze a lemon over the mixture and serve at room temperature.

Note: This tastes great if you make it a day ahead. Let the mixture sit in the fridge overnight and then take it out to bring it back to room temperature. Taste it again before serving, as you may not need to add the lemon juice. Serve with grilled fish, cold meats or warm crusty bread.

RADISH, CRAB AND BEETROOT SALAD

A lovely fresh salad with Blood-nourishing beetroot. Serve with a miso soup to add some digestive warmth.

Serves 2
200g white crab meat
2 beetroots, 1 of them yellow (if available)
white wine vinegar (if using yellow beetroot)
red wine vinegar
1 level tsp cayenne pepper
juice of 1 lime
1 tsp sea salt
1 pomegranate
1 small bunch of radishes
1 bag pea shoots

1. Preheat the oven to 160°C/310°F/gas mark 2½. Wash the beetroot, cut in half and place in a small ovenproof dish. Splash the white wine vinegar on the yellow beetroot, the red wine vinegar on the red and add water to a level halfway up the side of the dish. Cover and bake in the oven for 30 minutes, checking that the beetroot is soft in the centre with a sharp knife. Allow to cool.
2. In a bowl, mix the crab meat, cayenne pepper, lime juice and sea salt. Cut the pomegranate in half and tap the outside with a wooden spoon to release the seeds into a bowl. Slice the radish thinly. Add the radish, pea shoots and pomegranate seeds to the crab and toss, mixing well.
3. Scrape off the skin of the beetroot with a small knife and slice thinly. Lay in the centre of the plate, alternating the colours, and place the rest of the salad on top of the beetroot slices.

STICKY RICE AND PEACH (OR MANGO)

This comforting dessert is a perfect stomach tonic and is great for menstrual pain, and also for when you need something a little naughty, but oh so good. Life is nothing without a little sweetness.

Serves 2

¼ cup short-grain rice
1 cup coconut milk
100ml milk
1 vanilla pod
1 tbsp agave nectar syrup
zest from 1 orange
50ml cream
1 peach or mango (ripe and ready to eat)
½ tbsp brown sugar

1. Place the rice, coconut milk, milk, sugar, zest and vanilla pod (cut in half and with the seeds scraped a little to release the flavour) in a pan and bring to the boil over a medium heat.
2. Reduce the heat immediately, cover and allow to simmer, stirring every now and then to prevent it from sticking to the bottom and burning.
3. The rice is ready when it is soft to taste (brands of rice may vary a little so cook according to the packet instructions). Let it cool before adding the cream.
4. Place in two bowls and put in the fridge until you're ready to eat it, or you can serve it warm straight away. Serve topped with peach or mango slices and sprinkled with brown sugar.

Phase 2: Follicular

In this phase you should choose foods that support the gentle build-up of essential fluids and the maturation of the egg towards ovulation – these are Yin-nourishing foods. You should also include Blood-nourishing foods after your period so that you can use the full length of the cycle to build the quality of the endometrial lining. Avoid overstimulating foods (overly spicy foods, alcohol and caffeinated drinks) during this phase; coffee is a really bad idea. Hydrating foods, especially soups and herbal teas, are very helpful during this phase.

Yin-supporting foods:

- apples
- asparagus
- avocados
- bananas
- cheese
- clams
- crab
- duck
- eggs
- green beans
- honey
- kidney beans
- lemons
- malt
- mangoes
- milk
- nettles
- oysters
- peas
- pears
- pineapple
- pomegranates
- pork
- rabbit
- seaweed
- sesame
- spelt
- spinach
- sweet potatoes
- teas: dandelion, fennel, nettle
- tofu
- tomatoes
- watermelon
- wheat
- yams

Recipes

Chicken soup three ways

If you do nothing else from this book, start making chicken soup. As I see it, there are three ways to cook a chicken soup, all of which are deeply healing and nourishing. I think of these soups as being a bit like the stickers teachers put on homework when marking: Good, Very Good and Excellent. One is quick and fresh, one is slow and homely, and one leans on ancient traditions and healing. Take your pick!

GOOD

Chicken soup is often most needed when things are a bit tricky, time is tight, energy is low and we need a bit of soothing. This recipe is a quick fix for times such as these. Using good shop-bought chicken stock and some fresh herbs makes this a modern, warming and uplifting version of chicken soup.

Serves 4

rapeseed oil
2 onions, peeled and sliced
2 sticks celery, finely chopped (set aside the leaves)
2 carrots, peeled and finely diced
1.5 litres good chicken stock
small bunch of parsley, freshly chopped
small bunch of dill
celery leaves
salt and freshly ground black pepper

1. Heat a large saucepan over a medium heat and add the rapeseed oil, then the onions, celery and carrots and fry gently until they start to soften.
2. Add the chicken stock and bring your soup to a steady gentle boil. Taste and season with salt and pepper, then simmer for another 10 minutes until all the vegetables are cooked.
3. Stir in the herbs and serve in big bowls on laps.

VERY GOOD

Very good on many levels – this is a great way of using up leftovers from a roast-chicken dinner. Using roasted chicken adds a depth and sweetness to the soup.

Serves 4

the remains of a roast chicken
handful of chicken wings (if you have them)
2 leeks, washed and chopped into chunks
2 celery sticks, washed and chopped into chunks
a tomato or two
1 tsp peppercorns
small bunch of parsley
few sprigs of thyme
3 or 4 bay leaves

1. Take your largest pan and put the chicken leftovers into it: bones, meat and all the juices and jelly from the tray. Throw in the vegetables, herbs and peppercorns. Add enough water to just cover everything (about

2 litres). You might have to top up the liquid during cooking if it boils down too much.

2. Bring the whole lot to the boil and then turn the heat down – you want it just bubbling quietly. Leave to simmer gently for a couple of hours.

3. After a couple of hours, the broth will have turned a pale-golden tone. It should smell amazing. Next lift the bones out and strain the whole lot through a sieve into another pan.

4. Serve simply in a bowl, with a little bread if you want.

EXCELLENT

For when full soothing is needed. For this one you'll need a trip to your Chinese supermarket, or you could order some bits online. I use a whole chicken here and nourishing Chinese dates and balancing ginseng root. A healing bowl of soup.

Serves 4
1.2kg whole chicken
4 finger-sized pieces of fresh or dried ginseng root, washed
4 Chinese red dates
2 shallots, peeled and roughly chopped
thumb-sized piece of ginger, peeled and sliced
2 cloves garlic, washed and finely chopped
2 spring onions, washed

1. Place the chicken in a large soup pot (or clay pot), add enough water to cover it, then scatter in the ginseng, garlic, ginger and red dates and bring it to boil.

2. Simmer for over an hour, skimming off any white foam which rises to the top with a ladle.

3. Before serving, carefully remove the chicken from the pan and shred the meat. Divide the meat between four bowls, then ladle over the soup. Finish with a sprinkling of spring onions and some black pepper.

EGG DROP SOUP

This is a nourishing and simple soup that warms and protects. It is fresh and satisfying, helping to support this pre-ovulation phase.

Serves 2

groundnut or vegetable oil
thumb-sized piece of ginger, peeled and finely chopped
6 spring onions, trimmed and finely sliced
1 clove of garlic, peeled and finely chopped
500ml of good chicken or vegetable stock
½ tsp white pepper
1 tbsp cornflour
2 free-range eggs
250g baby spinach
soy sauce to serve

1. Heat a little oil in a saucepan, add the ginger, garlic and spring onions and sizzle over a medium heat for a couple of minutes until the ginger and garlic have started releasing their aromas.
2. Next add the stock and the white pepper and bring to the boil, then turn down to a simmer. Mix the cornflour with a tablespoon of cold water, then stir it into the soup and simmer for a couple of minutes until the soup begins to thicken very slightly.
3. Now crack the eggs into a little jug, add a couple of tablespoons of water and mix with a fork. Whisk your soup with your fork and very slowly pour in the egg mixture, whisking all the time to create little strands of egg. Once all the egg is added, throw in your spinach and allow it to wilt down for a minute or so.
4. Serve with soy sauce on the side, to be added to taste.

SWEET TOMATO POACHED BASS

The sweetness of the tomatoes is good for Blood Stagnation (page 244). The cinnamon and rosemary are warming, while lemon zest helps with digestion.

Serves 2

2 cloves of garlic, peeled and finely sliced
1 sprig of fresh rosemary

1 red chilli
1 400g tin chopped tomatoes
2 bass fillets
olive oil
small handful of capers
½ cinnamon stick
good pinch of dried oregano
extra-virgin olive oil, for garnishing
bunch of basil
1 lemon

1. Heat a large pan on a medium heat, and once it's hot add a swig of olive oil and the garlic, rosemary leaves and whole chilli. Cook for a couple of minutes until the garlic softens.
2. Next add the tomatoes and a can of water and bring to a simmer, then season well with salt and pepper. Lower the bass fillets into the sauce, pushing it down so the sauce covers the fish completely.
3. Place a lid on your pot and simmer for around 10 minutes until the bass is just cooked.
4. This is best eaten just warm, so allow it to cool a little – the flavours will mingle as it cools. Serve the fish with the basil torn over, topped with a drizzle of olive oil and a grating of lemon zest, plus warmed wedges of bread for mopping up the sauce.

Black sesame seeds

I am a big fan of the humble sesame seed, and if you can get your hands on the black variety that is even better. These small black seeds are a wonderful Blood tonic and easy to sprinkle on anything. They are the most Yin of all foods so have a positive influence on all the Yin fluids of the body and importantly the follicle fluid in which the follicle develops and which influences the final stages of development of the egg.

BLACK SESAME TAHINI

Makes a nice jarful
100g black sesame seeds
140g walnuts
sea salt
1 tbsp honey

1. In a pan roast the black sesame seeds over a medium heat for 5 to 10 minutes until fragrant. Pour the roasted seeds into a bowl. Now roast the walnuts in the pan until golden brown.
2. Add the roasted seeds and walnuts to a food processor with a good pinch of sea salt and a tablespoon of honey. Blitz for a couple of minutes until you have a smooth, loose paste (if you like a really fine tahini, grind the toasted nuts and seeds in a spice mill or pestle and mortar before blitzing).
3. Add your tahini to salad dressings, stir into hummus, or serve with yoghurt, peaches and honey for dessert.

HONEY AND BLACK SESAME SNAPS

Makes about 15 snaps
200g black sesame seeds
100g runny honey
1 tbsp coconut milk
sea salt

1. Preheat your oven to 180°C/350°F/gas mark 4. Place the black sesame seeds into a bowl with the runny honey, coconut milk and a pinch of sea salt. Mix it all together well.
2. Pile onto a greased baking sheet, flattening out the mixture with the back of a spoon (it will spread a little more in the oven), and bake for about 5 to 7 minutes.
3. Allow to cool before snapping into snack-sized pieces. These are also brilliant crumbled over fruit and yoghurt or mango sorbet for a quick dessert.

SUPER GREENS WITH BLACK SESAME

Serves 2
groundnut oil
2 handfuls long-stem broccoli
2 pak choi, quartered
2 handfuls edamame beans, shelled and cooked
1 clove of garlic, finely chopped
sesame oil
handful of black sesame seeds
juice of ½ lemon
tamari or soy sauce

1. Heat a wok or large frying pan until nice and hot. Add a glug of groundnut oil, then the broccoli, pak choi and edamame beans. Stir-fry for a couple of minutes, then add the garlic and a splash of sesame oil.
2. Remove from the heat and sprinkle with the black sesame seeds. Squeeze over the lemon juice and splash on some tamari or soy. Serves two as a light meal; you could add some noodles tossed in sesame oil if you are hungry.

SUPER BLACK SESAME RICE BOWL

Serves 4
200g short-grain brown rice
sea salt
2 sheets nori seaweed
juice of ½ lemon
juice of ½ orange
1 tsp honey
2 tbsp soy sauce
2 tbsp rice vinegar
1 pomegranate
1 avocado, chopped
bunch of coriander, chopped
2 handfuls black sesame seeds, toasted

1. Boil the rice in double the amount of water and a pinch of sea salt for 40 minutes until the grains are tender and all the water has been absorbed.
2. Toast the nori in a pan, then crumble into pieces.
3. Make the dressing: mix together the lemon juice, orange juice, honey, soy and rice vinegar.
4. Put the cooked rice in a bowl with the nori, the pomegranate seeds, avocado, coriander and toasted black sesame seeds. Pour over the dressing and serve just warm.

SPAGHETTI VONGOLE

This is a bit of an aphrodisiac; it's a light dish with a punch.

Serves 2

olive oil

300g fresh clams (the shells should mostly be closed; if some shells are slightly open, they should close when tapped)

200g spaghetti

1 small red chilli, finely chopped

1 clove garlic, crushed

butter – about a centimetre cubed

1 lime

sea salt

3 splashes of white wine

handful of coriander, chopped

1. Place some oil in a hot pan. Once the oil is hot, fry off the chilli and then add the clams. Cook for around two minutes before adding the garlic and continue to cook.
2. Season with salt and squeeze the lime over the clams. Cook until all the clams are open. Add the white wine (it should sizzle) and then lower the heat.
3. In the meantime, bring a pan of water to the boil and cook the spaghetti. A timer makes this job easier. Drain the pasta and add to the clams, tossing them around the pan for a couple of minutes to really coat the strands of spaghetti in the juices.
4. Taste and season if you need to. Remove from the heat and add the coriander. Place into a big serving bowl for sharing.

MARINATED TOFU

Tofu is easy on the digestive system and a good source of protein. This recipe nourishes your Qi, Blood and Yin and even Yang. It's a bit of a super-fertility recipe.

Serves 2

150g silken firm tofu (fresh)
1 tbsp chilli flakes
1 tbsp white sesame seeds
1 tbsp black sesame seeds
½ tbsp turmeric powder (or use fresh grated turmeric)
½ tbsp fennel seeds
½ tbsp mustard seeds
sesame or walnut oil
sea salt

1. Mix the seeds and spices together in a bowl.
2. Drain the tofu and cut into cubes. Add to the spices and toss gently in the bowl to make sure the tofu is coated well. Cover and leave in the fridge overnight.
3. To serve, drizzle with sesame or walnut oil and season with sea salt.

SUPERGREENS SALAD

This is best eaten just after your period. It's also excellent in between IVF cycles to help liver function. The idea with this salad is that nothing is cooked: instead, you mulch the greens with a little salt and lemon juice to give you maximum nutrients from all of these super nutrient-rich greens. Eat with a bowl of soup on the side.

Serves 2

good handful of watercress
good handful of kale
good handful of spinach
handful of bitter leaves, like dandelion or radicchio
handful of dried seaweed
juice of 1 lime
sea salt

100g sesame seeds, toasted
1 tbsp soy sauce
1 tbsp sesame oil
1 tbsp brown sugar
1 tbsp rice vinegar

1. First make your dressing by mixing the brown sugar into the rice vinegar until it dissolves. Then add all the rest of the ingredients and mix together.
2. Put the watercress, kale, spinach and bitter leaves into a bowl. Squeeze over the juice of the lime and sprinkle with a pinch of sea salt. Get your hands into the bowl and mulch the greens together, squashing and squeezing until the hardier greens have broken down.
3. Add the seaweed and sesame seeds and pour over the dressing. Serve in big bowls as a lovely energy-giving lunch.

Phase 3: Ovulation

Ovulation is a time when our Qi, or energy, needs to be supported. Opt for oats in the morning and eat lightly in the evening. Try simply grilled grapefruit topped with ginger, basil and brown sugar for a warming citrus treat.

Qi-supporting foods:

- almonds
- beef
- carrots
- cherries
- chicken
- chickpeas
- coconut
- dates
- eggs
- figs
- grapes
- ham
- lentils
- licorice
- mackerel
- milk
- millet
- molasses
- oats
- octopus
- pheasant
- potatoes
- quinoa
- rabbit
- rice
- sage
- sardines
- sweet potatoes
- shiitake mushrooms
- squash

- teas: digestive tea (caraway, dill, fennel seed and coriander seed), green tea
- tofu
- trout
- venison
- yams

Recipes

HERB MUFFINS

A healthy savoury treat, full of warming herbs.

Makes 12–16 muffins
310g plain flour
40g quick cooking oats or oat flour
1 tsp baking powder
1 tsp bicarbonate of soda
½ tsp salt
1 tsp fresh thyme
½ tsp fresh rosemary, finely chopped
¼ tsp fresh sage, finely chopped
370g courgettes, grated
135g pine nuts
50g parmesan or extra-mature cheddar, grated (plus a little more for garnishing)
170g butter, melted
2 eggs
zest of 1 lemon

1. Preheat the oven to 190°C/375°F/gas mark 5. Butter each muffin cup in your muffin pan and set aside.
2. In a bowl combine the flour, oats, baking powder, bicarbonate of soda and salt.
3. In a large mixing bowl whisk the eggs lightly with a fork, adding the herbs. Stir in the grated courgettes, followed by the melted butter. Stir the flour mixture into the courgette mixture, adding the pine nuts, lemon zest and cheese.
4. Spoon the mixture into the muffin cups, filling them completely, and sprinkle a little of the extra grated cheese on each. Bake on the middle rack for 30–40 minutes until they are golden brown and springy when you

press on them. (Please note that each oven is different and cooking times may vary accordingly.) Test with a thin skewer to make sure the muffins are cooked through – the skewer should come out clean when they are ready.

5. Let the muffin tin cool for 5 minutes and then remove the muffins and allow to cool on a wire rack for 15 minutes.

CARROT AND SQUASH SOUP WITH WARM SPICES AND FENNEL TOASTS

A vibrant sunset-orange soup with warm spices to aid digestion, excellent for Thinkers (see page 122). This is strongly supportive to the body's Yang and Qi, gently warming and tonifying. 'Tonifying' is a term I use all the time and is central to how I practise. It means to bring energy to something or to raise the energy of something; we could use it to describe a food or meal, but it can also apply to acupuncture treatment or exercise for example. Sometimes I look at a person and think 'this person is exhausted and needs tonifying'. Fennel is also excellent for relieving digestive Stagnation.

Serves 6
olive oil or rapeseed oil
1 large onion, peeled and finely chopped
2 sticks of celery, trimmed and chopped
2 cloves of garlic, peeled and finely chopped
1 tsp fennel seeds
1 tsp coriander seeds
1 tsp caraway seeds
5 cardamom pods
1 butternut squash, peeled, deseeded and roughly chopped
6 medium carrots, peeled and roughly chopped
1.5 litres of hot vegetable stock
6 slices sourdough bread
1 head of fennel, plus the leafy tops
1 lemon
sea salt
freshly ground black pepper

1. First heat up your biggest pan and add a good glug of olive or rapeseed oil. Add the chopped, onion, celery and garlic and sweat over a low heat for around 10 minutes.

2. Meanwhile, crush the cardamom seeds in a pestle and mortar until the pods have split, and remove the little seeds. Throw the pods away. Add all the remaining spices to the mortar and crush until you have a rough powder. Add this to the onions.

3. Continue to cook the onions for 10 minutes until they are soft and sweet. Next add the chopped squash, the carrots and the stock. Bring the whole lot to the boil, then turn the heat down to simmer and allow it to bubble away for about 40 minutes until the carrots and squash are soft and cooked through. Season with a good pinch of sea salt.

4. Remove the soup from the heat and use a hand blender to blitz the soup until it is lovely and smooth.

5. To make your toasts, finely shred or grate your fennel and put in a bowl with a pinch of sea salt, a pinch of black pepper, a good drizzle of olive oil and a squeeze of lemon. Use your hands to mix and squish all the flavours together. Toast the bread and drizzle with a bit more olive oil, then top with the fennel and serve with a bowl of bright, piping-hot soup.

PEARL BARLEY WITH ROASTED SWEET POTATO, ORANGE AND BITTER HERBS

Warm and filling, this is a proper nourisher. Eat it under a blanket on the sofa. Pearl barley provides a carbohydrate hit to calm and soothe; feel free to use other wholegrains, such as quinoa, farro or bulgur wheat. Sweet potato moves the Blood, while the bitter chicory and mint stimulate digestion, and finally sage and rosemary warm like a blanket. Perfect for supper or a packed lunch.

Serves 4
300g pearl barley
3 large sweet potatoes, peeled and roughly chopped into big chunks
2 sprigs of rosemary, chopped
sea salt and freshly ground black pepper
olive oil
handful of almonds
few sprigs of sage
100g parmesan, grated
1 orange
2 heads of red or white chicory, roughly chopped
small bunch of mint, chopped

1. Preheat your oven to 200°C/400°F/gas mark 6. Bring a pan of water to the boil and cook the pearl barley for 25 minutes until tender.
2. While the pearl barley is bubbling away, throw the sweet potatoes into a roasting tin with the rosemary, a good pinch of salt and pepper and a glug of oil, and roast in the oven for 35 minutes until soft and golden around the edges.
3. Put the almonds, sage, parmesan and zest and juice of half the orange into a food processor with a couple of good glugs of olive oil and a pinch of salt and pepper. Blitz until it looks like pesto. If you don't have a food processor, use a pestle and mortar to crush the nuts and sage, then add the other ingredients.
4. Once your pearl barley is cooked, drain well, then add to a big bowl with the chicory and mint and the roasted sweet potatoes. Drizzle over your pesto-like dressing and serve warm.

QUINOA SALAD

Quinoa is brilliant when you are trying to conceive and you can feel your Heart energy becoming a little depleted. It boosts the Qi of the whole body and is high in protein – really good protein that can improve embryo quality. Quinoa is very easy to cook. When cooked, the germ falls away and retains an ever-so-slight crunch, while the seed itself becomes tender and transparent. It has a light, delicate taste and is highly nutritious.

Serves 6

500g of uncooked quinoa
100g sun-blushed tomatoes, plus 2 tbsp of their oil
1 large onion, finely chopped
1 courgette, diced
1 clove of garlic, crushed
150g cooked chickpeas
2 tbsp toasted pumpkin seeds or pine nuts

1. Rinse the quinoa in cold running water and drain. Place in a saucepan with plenty of water, bring to the boil and simmer for 8 to 10 minutes. Drain well in a fine sieve and set aside.
2. Meanwhile, heat a little of the tomato oil in a large frying pan and fry the onions for 3 to 4 minutes, until they just start to colour. Add the

courgettes, garlic, chickpeas and chopped tomatoes and cook over a high heat until warmed through.

3. Stir the cooked quinoa through the vegetables and serve in warmed bowls. Sprinkle with toasted pumpkin seeds or pine nuts.

SPICY QUINOA AND VEGETABLES

This warming recipe is ideal for those who need a little heat in their bellies.

> **Serves 3–4**
> *200g uncooked quinoa*
> *200g mixed seasonal vegetables*
> *1 litre milk*
> *4 tbsp curry paste (I use Patak's vindaloo paste)*
> *1 large onion, sliced*
> *2 tbsp coriander or parsley, chopped*
> *two or three fresh chillies, chopped (optional)*

1. Rinse the quinoa in cold running water and drain, then set aside.
2. Heat a little oil in a large saucepan and gently fry the onion with the curry paste for about 5 minutes, stirring from time to time.
3. Meanwhile, wash and chop your vegetables.
4. Heat the milk in a separate small saucepan, being careful not to allow it to boil.
5. Add the vegetables and the quinoa to the curry and onion mix, then stir in the milk. Bring mixture to the boil and simmer gently for about 10 minutes, until the vegetables and quinoa are cooked.
6. Serve in warmed bowls and garnish with chopped coriander or parsley.

TABOULEH

This recipe can be made with the traditional bulgur wheat or with quinoa. Parsley is an excellent Blood tonic and helps to drain excess fluid from the body. This is also the perfect remedy for those who are feeling a bit 'stuck'.

> **Serves 6–8**
> *480ml chicken stock*
> *170g bulgur wheat or quinoa*
> *⅓ cucumber, peeled, deseeded and roughly chopped*

3 ripe but firm tomatoes, peeled, deseeded and chopped
large bunch of flat-leaf parsley, finely chopped
large bunch of curly parsley, finely chopped
large bunch of mint, finely chopped
6 spring onions or 3 small shallots, finely sliced
freshly ground black pepper, to taste
2 large, juicy lemons
120ml olive oil
1 tsp sea salt
1 tsp ground cumin

1. Bring the stock to a boil, add the bulgur or quinoa, stir well, then cover. Cook for about 15–20 minutes, stirring occasionally, until plumped up (refer to packet instructions if necessary). Drain off any excess liquid, fluff up the grains with a fork, then set aside to cool.
2. Put the cucumber and tomato in a bowl, along with the parsley, mint and onion.
3. In a jar with a lid, combine the lemon juice, olive oil, salt and cumin, shaking vigorously until it is emulsified.
4. Add the bulgur or quinoa to the bowl (it's fine if it's still a bit warm), add all of the dressing and stir well. Season with fresh pepper and salt if needed. Let the tabouleh stand for a couple of hours before serving, or leave in the fridge overnight (bring up to room temperature to serve); the flavours will meld together well as it stands.

PICKLED CABBAGE

This recipe is warming and moving, dispersing Stagnation and supporting the liver. Cabbage is amazing for its Heat-resolving anti-inflammatory effects.

Serves 6–8 (as a side)
6 crushed cardamom pods
1½ tsp clove powder (or 6 cloves)
200ml apple cider vinegar
200ml umeboshi plum vinegar
800ml water
1 tbsp sea salt (smoked if available)
1 tsp coriander seeds, crushed
1 white cabbage

1. Place all of the ingredients except the cabbage in a pan and bring to the boil.
2. Reduce the heat and let simmer for 3 or 4 minutes.
3. Slice the cabbage finely, and then pour over the pickling liquid. Allow to cool and then refrigerate until use. This will keep for about a month.

Phase 4: Luteal

This is the incubation phase and so we include plenty of warming, Yang-supporting foods.

Yang-supporting foods:

- anchovies
- aniseed
- basil
- cardamom
- chestnuts
- cinnamon
- cloves
- fennel seeds
- fenugreek seeds
- garlic
- ginger
- kidneys
- lamb
- nutmeg
- pistachios
- prawns
- quinoa
- rosemary
- sage
- star anise
- teas: sweet chai, PMTea (see recipes below)
- thyme
- trout
- venison
- walnuts

Recipes

SWEET CHAI

Serves 2
350ml water
½ stick cinnamon
8 cardamom pods
6 cloves
½ centimetre fresh ginger, sliced
150ml milk
2 tsp honey
3 tsp Darjeeling tea leaves

1. Heat the water in a saucepan, add the cinnamon, cardamom, cloves and ginger, and bring to the boil. Lower the heat and simmer with the lid on for 10 minutes.
2. Add the milk and honey and continue to simmer for a minute.
3. Remove from the heat and add the tea leaves. Allow to steep for a couple of minutes.

PMTEA (FIG, ORANGE ZEST, FENNEL AND CAMOMILE TEA)

A real rescue remedy of a tea, it gently moves Qi and calms the mind. This tea could calm a banshee.

> **Makes a big potful**
> *1.5 litres water*
> *6 dried figs*
> *1 tbsp camomile flowers (or 2 camomile teabags)*
> *1 tsp fennel seeds*
> *zest of 1 orange, peeled into strips with a veg peeler*

1. Put all the ingredients in a big pan and cover with the water. Bring to the boil and simmer for 20 minutes or so until the liquid has reduced by about a third.
2. Strain, keep warm and sip throughout the day.

SPICED PORRIDGE

1. The night before, boil some water and add a few strips of orange peel, a couple of cloves, cardamom pods and a star anise (if you have it). After steeping for a few minutes, pour the liquid over your usual portion of porridge oats in a bowl.
2. Let this stand overnight. In the morning simply heat up in a pan. Serve with fresh or soft dried figs and, if you like, a spoonful of natural yoghurt (if you tend towards feeling Heat).

MINESTRONE

There are many ways to make minestrone, and I rarely make it the same way twice. The only rule I stick to is always using vegetables that are in season. For instance, in winter I use cabbage, and in spring I use asparagus, peas and fennel. In summer and as autumn approaches I use carrots, courgettes and celery. Minestrone can be a whole meal if you want it to be, but this particular version is fairly light, as I have replaced the traditional bacon and pasta and used aduki beans in their place. Aduki beans are great for draining Dampness from the body. I also sprinkle over a few green nori flakes for extra nourishment.

Amaranth and quinoa are both exceptionally high in protein, making them unusually nutritious. Amaranth is slightly cool in nature, whereas quinoa is slightly warm. So if you are a Hot type, amaranth is slightly better for you; Cold types should choose quinoa.

Serves 6
olive oil
1.5 litres good chicken or vegetable stock
1 large onion, peeled and finely chopped
1 small leek, finely sliced
8 large tomatoes, blanched, deseeded and chopped
4 cloves of garlic, peeled and crushed
2 carrots, finely chopped
2 sticks of celery, finely chopped
110g green beans, finely chopped
1 small red pepper, deseeded and finely chopped
1 small courgette, finely chopped
small bunch of flat-leaf parsley, chopped
225g cooked aduki beans
1 tbsp dried green nori flakes to garnish
6 tbsp of fresh pesto
110g precooked quinoa or amaranth (optional)

1. Blanch the tomatoes, remove the seeds and chop.
2. Cook the onion and leeks in the oil in a large casserole or pan over a medium heat for about 10 minutes, until the onions are transparent.
3. Add the garlic and cook for 1 minute.

4. Add the tomatoes and stock and the rest of the prepared vegetables, leaving the courgettes until the very end as they only take a minute to cook. Bring to the boil, reduce the heat to low, cover and simmer gently for about 10 minutes, until the vegetables are tender but still with a slight bite to them.
5. Stir in the aduki beans, courgettes and chopped parsley and quinoa or amaranth (if using), bring back to the boil and simmer for about a minute.
6. Taste and season if necessary. Serve in big bowls with a generous tablespoon of pesto and a sprinkling of green nori flakes.

PESTO

I usually make pesto using a pestle and mortar, but do use a food processor if you prefer. If using a food processor, put in all the ingredients except the oil and process to a paste. Gradually trickle in the oil to give a creamy consistency. Yang-supporting walnuts make a great alternative to pine nuts.

Makes 6 tablespoons
25g basil
15g pine nuts
25g parmesan
50ml extra-virgin olive oil
1 or 2 cloves of garlic
¼ tsp sea salt
squeeze of lemon juice

Strip the leaves off the basil, place them in a mortar and pound with a little sea salt. Add the garlic and pine nuts and keep pounding until you have a paste. Work in the parmesan, constantly grinding and pounding. Add a squeeze of lemon juice and enough olive oil to give a creamy consistency.

SLOW ROASTED LEG OF LAMB

In fertility terms, warmth has always been considered to be an important factor in helping to incubate an embedding embryo in the luteal phase of the cycle. As the saying goes: 'You can't grow a baby in a fridge'. So warming comfort foods are important at any time in the cycle, but particularly for Cold types in the luteal (pre-menstrual) phase. Lamb and rosemary are the greatest of companions in the kitchen. Lamb is considered the most heating of meats, which is why it is often served with cooling mint or yoghurt. In this recipe we are going all out for warmth.

Serves 6-8
1 leg of lamb
4–6 large potatoes, scrubbed and thickly sliced
1 onion, thinly sliced
6–8 cloves of garlic, peeled and sliced
few sprigs of rosemary
about 600ml stock (use half stock and half dry white wine if you prefer)

1. Preheat the oven to 200°C/400°F/gas mark 6. Make little incisions all over the lamb and push the slivers of garlic into each hole, followed by a little sprig of rosemary. Season the lamb with salt and pepper.
2. Grease the casserole with a little butter and layer the potatoes and onions at the bottom of the dish, seasoning with a little salt and pepper. Pour the stock over the top of the potatoes to just cover them and sit the lamb on top of the potatoes.
3. Pop the casserole into the oven and roast for about 15–20 minutes until the casserole and its contents are piping hot.
4. Turn the oven temperature down to 140°C/275°F/gas mark 1 and continue to roast for about 4 hours, until the lamb flakes away from the bone and the potatoes are crisp on the top and moist underneath.

ROASTED SQUASH WITH RATATOUILLE AND CHESTNUTS

2 small butternut squash
1 clove of garlic, crushed
3 tbsp olive oil
pinch of chilli flakes
1 small courgette, cut into 2-centimetre pieces
1 small red pepper, cut into 2-centimetre pieces
2 small red onions, chopped
200g cherry tomatoes
1–2 tbsp olive oil
1 tbsp fresh thyme or basil

50g whole cooked chestnuts, chopped
100g goat's cheese, cut into small pieces
1 tbsp fresh breadcrumbs
1 tbsp fresh parsley, chopped
1 tbsp parmesan, grated

1. Preheat the oven to 200°C/400°F/gas mark 6. Cut the squash in half and scoop out the seeds (keep the seeds for later). Cut criss-cross patterns over the cut side of each squash (I find that the deeper you make the cuts in the squash, the faster it cooks).
2. Mix the garlic, olive oil and chilli together and brush the mixture over the flesh of the squash. Pop in the oven and bake for 30–40 minutes, until the flesh is tender.
3. To make the ratatouille filling, put all the prepared vegetables into a roasting tin, add the herbs and drizzle with olive oil, season and roast for about 20 minutes. Add the cherry tomatoes and cook for another 10 minutes.
4. Add the chopped chestnuts and goat's cheese to the ratatouille mix. Arrange the ratatouille mix over the cooked squash halves. Mix together the breadcrumbs, parsley and parmesan and scatter over the top, then bake for a further 10 minutes until golden and bubbling.
5. Serve hot with a generous helping of hummus.

Note: Use vacuum-packed whole cooked chestnuts if fresh ones are not available. You can vary the ingredients for the filling using different vegetables, nuts and cheese; pine nuts work particularly well.

STICKY GINGER MOLASSES CAKE

Sticky and moreish, a little wedge of this homemade treat will provide a more balanced boost when you hit an energy low. The ginger helps with digestion, while the warming spices soothe. Iron-rich molasses bolsters your energy supply and provides a less refined sweet hit.

Makes 12 slices
300g plain flour
1 tsp ground cinnamon
½ tsp ground cloves
200g light brown sugar

300ml molasses
2 large eggs
250ml groundnut oil
2 tsp baking powder
100ml boiling water
100g fresh ginger, peeled and finely chopped
2 apples, roughly grated

1. Grease a 20-centimetre round spring-form cake tin. Preheat the oven to 180°C/350°F/gas mark 4.
2. In a large bowl sift together the flour, cinnamon and cloves.
3. In another bowl beat the molasses, sugar, eggs and oil with an electric hand whisk for a couple of minutes until lighter in colour and all mixed together. Next add the flour and spice mixture and mix with a spoon until just combined.
4. Now stir the baking soda into the water and, wasting no time, quickly add this to the mixture along with the chopped ginger and grated apple. Mix together until just blended. Pour the mixture into the prepared tin and level out.
5. Bake in a preheated oven for around an hour; test by inserting a toothpick – it should come out clean. If the top browns too quickly, cover loosely with foil and return to the oven.
6. Cool on a rack before cutting into snack-sized wedges.

CRANACHAN

My take on the classic Scottish dessert. Oats, walnuts and spices all aid the luteal phase. This is a lighter take on cranachan, using yoghurt instead of cream. Cranachan is a killer dessert, but could easily be eaten at breakfast time too.

Serves 4
40g rolled oats
pinch of cinnamon
good grating of fresh nutmeg
100g walnuts, crumbled
200g raspberries
200ml of natural or Greek yoghurt
2 tbsp runny honey

1. Preheat the oven to 200°C/400°F/gas mark 6. Spread your oats and crumbled walnuts over a baking sheet with the spices, then toast in the hot oven for 5 to 10 minutes until they smell sweet and nutty.
2. Crush half the raspberries with a fork, then fold these into the yoghurt and stir in the runny honey. Add the remaining whole raspberries, then fold in the toasted oats and spoon into 4 little glasses and serve.

Fertility superfoods

Flax seeds

Flax seeds are high in essential omega-3 and omega-6 fatty acids, which are helpful for balancing hormones. They also contain B vitamins, magnesium, manganese and phytoestrogens, which help block harmful xenoestrogens (compounds found in things like insecticides and pesticides that mimic oestrogen in the body and so can disrupt hormonal balance). The best way to absorb the nutrients from flax seeds is to freshly grind them each day in your spice grinder and add a tablespoon to your porridge. Pumpkin seeds are also a particular favourite of mine.

Almonds

Of all the nuts I would favour the almond, which in Ayurvedic medicine is considered the finest of nuts since it builds *ojas* (Jing) and is therefore restorative for the reproductive system. Almonds are best cracked yourself and blanched in boiling water so that the skins are removed, as these are hard on the digestion. Blanching will also begin the process of germination if left overnight to soak, which will improve digestibility. Warning: if you tend to produce phlegm easily, eat almonds sparingly.

Seaweed and nettles

These are the supreme Blood builders, being high in iron and folic acid. In the spring, fresh nettle tea is delicious: just snip off the young tops and infuse in boiling water, as when making fresh mint tea. Nettle broth is very fortifying: simmer nettle tops in stock with chopped onions, celery and carrots and add a dash of tamari before serving. Seaweed is also making a well-deserved comeback. Wakame chopped into thin strips and added to an omelette along with sesame seeds is great served with a dipping soy or sweet chilli sauce for a fertility superfood lunch. Other greens, like rocket and watercress, are also well worth including in your diet in salads, or watercress is great made into soup with a little sour cream and nutmeg to warm the body.

Sesame seeds

These little seeds really are miraculous in their health-giving potential. Not only are they the most Yin of foods, they are also said to provide energy, a tranquil frame of mind and slow the ageing process. Use sesame oil for salads – it is tasty and very digestible – and sprinkle sesame seeds on vegetables, rice, salads, soups. *Functional Foods from the East* recommends '3g but preferably 10g every day of sesame seeds and oil for promotion of health and prosperity of people throughout the entire world'.

Alfalfa sprouts

These are bursting with vitality and are also alkaline, so they help to prevent too much acidity developing in the body – acidity is not helpful when it comes to fertility, particularly the production of cervical mucus. They are perfect for adding to salads or grains. Alfalfa sprouts are full of enzymes which help assimilate proteins, fats and carbohydrates.

Warning: Alfalfa sprouts are full of the amino acid canavanine, so should be avoided by those who have rheumatoid arthritis.

Quinoa

Quinoa is a great tonic for Qi, particularly helpful around the middle part of the menstrual cycle. It is high in good protein – great for embryo quality. If you do not currently eat quinoa, do try to include some regularly into your diet. I love quinoa and use it often; it's a great alternative to rice, pasta or potatoes. I use it to stuff roasted peppers and also as an alternative to bulgur wheat in tabouleh. Quinoa is very easy to cook (see recipes on pages 85 and 86). Barley and buckwheat are also well worth a try; and although rice gets a bad press, I am a fan and I think it is fine to include once a week in the diet. Risotto is a favourite of mine and this can be made either in the traditional way or with barley. Made with fresh chicken stock and finished with a knob or butter and a sprinkling of parmesan, there is no better comfort food. Don't stress about using butter in cooking: we need fat in our diets, and life without butter is a dull life indeed in my book.

Raspberries

The raspberry is my favourite berry by far, but any berry is good for you (although I sometimes think blueberries taste a little mouldy, so be sure to wash them well). Raspberries build the Blood and are very regulating for the menstrual cycle. Raspberry leaf tea is also a wonderful tonic and good to drink for all women who are trying to conceive, as it is thought to regulate the hormones. In terms of Chinese medicine, raspberries tonify Liver and Kidney energy, which are the organs most associated with conception. Eat raspberries in any way you like, but avoid the old-fashioned approach of sprinkling with sugar. My IVF fail-safe for raspberries is a smoothie made with whey protein, flax seeds and raspberries (see page 219).

Organic chicken and eggs

Nothing could be simpler than a roast chicken. It's so easy and so good, and one roast chicken stretches to about three meals in our house. Roast chicken is high in protein and low in fat (as long as you don't eat the skin), and there is so much you can do with it. You can roast it whole or cut it up and make it into a stew. You can use the entire chicken to make an incredible soup – or just the bones if you prefer to eat the chicken first. Buy the best quality chicken you can, eat the whole lot, then boil the bones for soup. You will never look back. If there is only one piece of advice you ever follow from this book, it should be: boil your chicken bones to make chicken soup. Eggs too are a powerhouse of goodness and so versatile. Eating three or four eggs per week provides a great Blood and Yin tonic.

Cabbage

This has long been considered to possess healing qualities in many countries, probably due to its anti-inflammatory effects. Cabbage is a cruciferous vegetable that is packed with antioxidants, which fight free radicals, and a phytonutrient which helps with oestrogen metabolism (this may be helpful in preventing endometriosis and fibroids). I was raised in Germany (my father was in the British army) and so grew up on sauerkraut, which I find very healing – it improves gut flora and rejuvenates and soothes the entire digestive tract. Bubble and squeak is a favourite in my house. Cabbage goes very well with fennel and carrot, and makes a great weight-loss soup.

Cinnamon

An amazing little spice, which I use frequently. If you struggle to see its use for anything other than sweet foods, look no further than the great Yotam Ottolenghi, who uses it in much of his Middle Eastern fusion-style cooking. Cinnamon is a Yang tonic, gently warming the body and activating the Qi. Adding cinnamon to a high-carbohydrate meal can help reduce the subsequent peak in blood sugar levels and so improve insulin sensitivity, which also makes it helpful for PCOS (see page 194). An interesting way to use cinnamon and other warm spices such as nutmeg and ginger is with sweet potato or yam. It may sound strange, but the drying, warming nature of the spices works very well to counterbalance the moist, sweet nature of the vegetable.

Oats

A great Qi tonic, oats gently warm the body and are particularly helpful for the thyroid and libido. They also nourish the all-important Jing of the body, making them a superfood in my book. Porridge with cinnamon and flax seeds makes for the ultimate power fertility breakfast, but don't limit oats to porridge. Put a handful in soups, or mix with sesame seeds and dip raw chicken pieces in egg and then into the oaty-sesame mix before frying to make healthy nuggets. Try cooking oats in chicken stock to make an oaty version of risotto. Or make a savoury crumble as a topping for a midweek vegetable bake (mix together 100g oats, 50g almond flakes, a little butter or olive oil, sea salt and a herb of your choice – I like fresh parsley).

Royal jelly

This is a menstrual regulator and can increase sperm count in men.

Algae

Algae contains high levels of amino acids, minerals, nutrients and live enzymes, in particular the B vitamins, which are good for fertility.

Chlorella

This is a single-celled fresh water algae and is an amazing supplement. It is known for its high levels of B12 and its Blood nourishing abilities.

Goji berries (wolfberries)

These berries are thought to improve sperm count in men, while in women they promote follicular growth and help ovulation. You can snack on them or cook with them, just as you would with raisins.

IN PRAISE OF THE ONE-POT MEAL

Cooking a number of ingredients together in one pot (soups, congee, casseroles and stews) is both convenient and a healthy way to eat. Often the food is cooked in the pot in the oven slowly, so that the ingredients become slightly broken down and the nutrients release themselves into the fluid. It is so much better in the winter than living off salads and raw food, which are cold and hard to digest. This way of eating is particularly good for those who have a weak digestion and are short on time. Bring back the slow cooker, I say!

THE BENEFITS OF TEA

There have been many hundreds of research papers published on the health-giving benefits of tea. Tea is said to be helpful for benefiting digestion and lifting the mood, and some studies have demonstrated a reduction in the risk of developing coronary heart disease, improved healthy bones, gums and teeth, a reduction in the risk of breast cancer in younger women, and protection against Alzheimer's and depression in the elderly. These benefits are down to the antioxidant catechins found in tea, as well as tannin, caffeine, theanine, theobromine and theophylline – together they promote relaxation and act as a smooth muscle relaxant. There has been a limited study that suggests drinking large amounts of green tea may block the absorption of folic acid, but a cup or two hasn't been shown to have any such effect. If you are taking a folic acid supplement, wait a few hours afterwards before drinking green tea.

Supplements

Even if you eat a well-balanced healthy diet, it is thought by many nutritionists that our foods can be lacking in certain nutrients. Here are the extra food supplements that are recommended for fertility:

- Multi-vitamins provide a combination of essential vitamins and minerals. It is a good idea to go for one specifically designed for women (and the same goes for men).
- A flax seed and/or fish oil supplement is good for general health.
- Vitamin C is an excellent antioxidant that may also be good for sperm count and quality.
- Zinc may help with both female and male fertility, plus it has been shown to support normal cell division in a new embryo.
- Folic acid promotes normal embryo development and is taken to prevent spina bifida. Any woman considering having a baby is advised to take folic acid.
- B vitamins: vitamin B12 helps with the absorption of folic acid, and a vitamin B12 deficiency has been proven to be a potential factor that affects ovulation. Vitamin B6 has been shown to boost female fertility.
- Iron. You may be advised by your doctor or a nutritionist that you need an iron supplement if you show signs of anaemia.
- Vitamin D: the easiest way to get your daily dose of vitamin D is to go outside for 20 minutes a day. There have been studies to show that this vitamin may help to balance sex hormones in women and improve sperm count in men.[47]

VITAMIN D

Studies have consistently shown that there is a high prevalence of vitamin D deficiency in Western populations, and even more for highly pigmented (darker) skin.

It has been consistently demonstrated that those who are deficient in vitamin D have an increased risk of pregnancy complications such as pre-eclampsia, low birth weight and pre-term delivery, so it is sensible to boost your vitamin D intake prior to conception.

Studies have shown a possible relationship between vitamin D supplementation and the improvement in symptoms of PCOS (see page 194), and a possible link between vitamin D and AMH levels. In a study of the over-40s there was a direct correlation between AMH levels and vitamin D.[48]

CHAPTER FIVE
FERTILITY IN THE GYM

The right kind of exercise, just like the right kind of food, can help to support normal female body function and is one of the core foundations for good health. Good exercise is an important building block for fertility and pregnancy, just as the wrong kind, like the wrong kind of food, can sometimes be detrimental.

Exercise is vital for our general health, wellbeing and fertility. Numerous studies confirm that many aspects of our health can improve through correct exercise and that a lack of exercise can be a cause of disease. So is all exercise good – is it as simple as that? Well, not quite, as not all exercise is equal.

The Royal College of Obstetricians and Gynaecologists give suggestions for exercise that is safe to do when you are pregnant, but there is little advice available about how much exercise to do while you are trying to get pregnant. Given that for two weeks of the month it is possible that you might be pregnant (while you're waiting to see if your period arrives), it stands to reason that if the right kind of exercise is a consideration during pregnancy, it is worth thinking about while trying to conceive too. Regular, moderate exercise has been shown to reduce oxidative stress and ageing.[49]

The research can be a little confusing and often conflicting, and as a result many women are not sure what to do for the best. Weight and body fat are significant; for instance, the NHS refuses IVF to women who have a high BMI (over 25 is considered overweight and 30 obese). I see women in my own practice who benefit greatly from gradually becoming more active and gently losing weight.

Recent studies now also demonstrate that it is women with low body fat (a BMI of under 18) who have worse outcomes in IVF. I frequently see women who are committed to wanting a baby but who are also committed to being thin, and so will work out quite obsessively in the gym and go on restrictive diets. By doing this they are running the risk of affecting their fertility. Research shows that for some women the body may not have enough energy to support both hard workouts and getting pregnant.[50] As my friend and psychologist Adriana Giotta puts it: 'In our world women are not often encouraged to just be. Each woman is unique and as such possesses her own body shape. Why try to all be the same? Let's see our body for what it actually is: a precious but simple container for our life force.'

Helping patients to feel good about themselves and to believe in their body's ability to conceive is an important consideration in fertility treatment. Fertility patients can start to lose faith in their bodies. As my colleague Tim Weeks, a fitness trainer, says: 'Unlock someone's belief, and they enter a whole new world.'

THE RIGHT KIND OF EXERCISE

Although there is plenty of information out there on exercise, much of it is very generic and does not necessarily consider the ultimate goal of the patient who is trying to conceive. Patients frequently ask me questions like: 'How much exercise can I do?', 'What sort of exercise should I choose?' and 'What intensity is right?' The answer to these questions is that it very much depends on who is asking the question. There is no one-size-fits-all approach. The type, amount and intensity of exercise will depend on how fit you are already and what you want to achieve. A woman who wants to conceive may need to shift her focus away from striving for a red-carpet body if her ultimate aim is to be pregnant.

EXERCISING TO EXHAUSTION

A thirty-four-year-old woman came to see me to help her conceive. She had been trying for several months and her periods had become irregular. She did not appear to be underweight, but she looked exhausted and was working long hours. I examined her tongue and was shocked to see it looked like the tongue of a woman in her menopause. Because her tongue looked unusual, I asked her if she was sweating abnormally. Eventually we worked out that she was going three times a week to a hot yoga class, designed to make you sweat. I could see from her tongue that this was having a detrimental effect on her: she was losing far too many fluids, which was causing her to feel exhausted and giving her the appearance (in terms of her fertility) of a menopausal woman. I should add here that this level of activity would not necessarily be quite so detrimental to everyone, although I do think it is too extreme for most women wanting to conceive. My patient changed her exercise schedule and gave up the hot yoga, continued with acupuncture and conceived within two menstrual cycles.

Here's the truth: exercise doesn't have to be hard or painful for it to make a big difference to your body or your health. If you ever feel the day after a workout or exercise class as though every muscle in your body has the flu, you are actually dehydrated. If specific muscles are feeling the burn, that's good – you are working a particular area well – but that fluey feeling is toxins running through your body, which aren't good for you at all. So think quality, not quantity, when it comes to exercise.

DO YOU NEED TO 'RESTORE' OR TO 'GET MOVING'?

There are two main types of exercise we will focus on, the objective being a healthy body plus healthy fertility. The first kind will restore the body when you are Deficient, while the second kind will get you moving to disperse Stagnation. Yoga (not the hot type!) and Qi Gong, for example, are restorative exercises that will help to build up your energy reserves and your stamina, whereas jogging, a spinning class, Zumba or Body Pump will get your blood pumping, dispersing Stagnation by helping to get energy flowing around the body.

The best person to determine what is best for you is you. If you have never done any exercise in your life, you should make sure you walk whenever you can and fit some movement into your day (like walking up the escalator on your commute or getting some fresh air every lunchtime). I promise that to do anything will be better than doing nothing. You can start with brisk walking. Many women are fans of either yoga (see below) or Pilates. But if you are a marathon runner, it will be more a case of understanding how to relax your training regime a bit without feeling you are getting slow or lazy. Perhaps the answer will be to add some yoga into your week rather than running every day, especially during your period.

It is vital to try to develop your own wisdom about when your body needs to move, and when it needs to rest and recuperate. So if you go to workout classes, for example, work at your own pace. When we sweat too much we may lose precious fluids (Yin) vital to our fertility. Men need to sweat because they do not have a menstrual cycle through which they can lose excess heat or toxins. It is important that you don't feel like you have been hit by a bus the day after exercising, as this is often due to overexerting when your system is feeling Stagnated. You might feel great just after your run or class, but really struggle for a day or even longer afterwards. So get to know what forms of exercise feel like they put energy into your tank and which are depleting. If you are ill, let your body rest and recover sufficiently, allow your energy reserves to build up gently rather than sweating things out in the gym.

EXERCISING THROUGH THE CYCLE

Phase 1: During your period

Gentle exercise is good to encourage Blood flow, but no swimming or anything too excessive. This might seem a tad old-fashioned, but bear with me! During the course of your period, the channels or meridians of the body are thought to be 'open', or more susceptible to external influence. Swimming potentially exposes women to Cold and Damp entering the body and disrupting the menses. I find this particularly true in young women, so caution is best taken early in life not to allow Cold and Damp to develop. Try to avoid swimming on the heaviest days of your cycle and keep exercise to a minimum. Staying warm and drying yourself adequately is crucial.

Phase 2: Follicular

It is generally fine to exercise how you like at this time, but remember that you are growing follicles and building Blood – so keep things steady and not excessive.

Phase 3: Ovulation

Activity and movement is important to keep the Qi activated in the pelvic cavity. Ten minutes of gentle rebound exercise (such as on a mini trampoline) is perfect to get the Qi flowing without depleting it.

Phase 4: Luteal

Immediately after ovulation, movement is good to help with free passage through the Fallopian tubes. If you are trying for a baby, calm things down about eight days after ovulation to encourage the implantation phase. If you know you aren't pregnant, exercise throughout the luteal phase is helpful to move Qi and Blood.

FERTILITY YOGA

Exercise isn't just about getting stronger and leaner; it can also be about stretching, movement, calming, preserving and releasing energy. That is why yoga is so aligned with fertility, because it helps with all of these things. As yoga expert Uma Dinsmore-Tuli says in her book *Womb Yoga* (see Resources): 'Yoga is all about refining awareness of body, mind, breath, emotions and energies . . . In the yogic anatomy of the energy body, the Womb is the seat of creativity, fertility and capacity to nurture and grow new life, new ideas – to manifest.'

Like myself, Uma believes that the intense heat and speed of hot yoga may have a drying effect, which for some women may deplete Yin (vital energies) and so compromise fertility.[51] The gentler form of Hatha yoga is particularly good if you are a beginner, and complements what we are trying to achieve with diet, the mind and understanding our body in relation to our fertility health. It was developed in India in the fifteenth century and is still the most popular form of yoga today. Its main aim is to develop balance between body and mind, to improve flexibility and strength and simply promote health and wellbeing. According to Uma, it is worth being aware that practising inversions in Hatha yoga during your period may lengthen the time you bleed.

QI GONG

Qi Gong, like yoga, is an excellent fertility exercise. It creates a flow of energy (Qi) around your body, bringing calmness and energy to both the body and the mind. It can be practised at home alone or at a class. It is a Chinese practice which involves slow movements combined with breathing techniques.

THE RIGHT TIME FOR EXERCISE

Pounding it out in the gym at the end of a long, hard day's work might make you feel good straight afterwards, because you'll be moving any Stagnation out of the body. But if you then feel shattered the day after, it's a sign that you were working out on empty and now your body is feeling Deficient. As with everything, it's crucial with exercise to get to know your own body and listen to how it responds to different types of exercise and exercising at different times of the day. Lots of people find swimming in the morning really sets them up for the day, giving them a good appetite and enabling them to focus on the day's work ahead; while others prefer the relaxation of a swim at the end of the day. Listen to your body and you will get to know what's best for you.

We don't tend to think of exercise in terms of how it might relate to the seasons, but our bodies do tend to feel different and have varied amounts of energy as the seasons change. In winter we instinctively want to conserve our energy, while in the spring we feel full of so much potential, so much more get-up-and-go. By the end of the year, with the culmination of the Christmas holidays for so many of us, we will often feel pretty exhausted or even stressed out. And then we try to hit the ground running in the New Year, with endless resolutions, just when our immune system is at its lowest. Ideally, we should take things nice and easy in the first couple of months of the year and then just as nature begins to wake up, so too should we nourish our bodies with more energetic exercise, especially outside whenever possible.

DON'T LET YOUR WORKOUT STRESS YOU OUT

- Gentle, rhythmic exercises like yoga and Qi Gong are great for releasing blocked energy and tension, rather than always thrashing it out in the gym. Movement and breathing come into sync with each other, and you can lose yourself in the flow.
- Just ten minutes of exercise will significantly increase your sense of get-up-and-go.
- Exercise outside and you will boost your daily levels of vitamin D at the same time.
- Do what feels right to you. If you're feeling happy but chatty, maybe a silent yoga class isn't what you need today. On the other hand, if your nerves are on edge from a hectic day at work, resist the temptation to sweat it out in a high-octane class and go for something more restorative, like a swim or a stretch class. Burning out in the gym will only heighten your stress levels.

CHAPTER SIX
FERTILITY IN THE BEDROOM

For to the bee a flower is a fountain of life – and to the flower a bee is a messenger of love – and to both, bee and flower, the giving and receiving of pleasure is a need and an ecstasy.

Khalil Gibran

In the 1950s, sex was a good option of an evening when we had little to distract us. Now we can choose to watch TV until late, use computers to catch up on work we didn't manage to finish in the day, and there is often little distinction between work and home life. So sex can come quite low down on the list of priorities, particularly if both partners are working.

It is not uncommon to see couples who have dramatically changed their lifestyles, are abstaining from alcohol, eating 'all the right foods', doing the right amount of exercise but having very little sex, or just a couple of well-timed baby-making sessions diarized into the month with precision. I would much prefer to see couples be more relaxed about diet and lifestyle issues and have more sex. As I said to one couple: 'Diet may make a difference and so might feeling relaxed, but the one thing we know for sure is that having sex will increase your chances of conception.' It sounds obvious, but you would be amazed at how often this is overlooked.

Until fairly recently the subject of sex was barely touched on in most GP consultations about fertility. I know people who have been offered IVF but never actually asked about their sex life (except maybe on a form). A couple

I saw recently were offered IVF; they had not actually had sex in six months – no one had bothered to discuss this as an issue.

There are a number of physical and psychological factors that may affect your sex life:

- Relationship problems can affect your sex life a great deal. It can be very beneficial to seek counselling from an organization such as Relate (see Resources). Perhaps resentment or blame have built up, for instance. It's vital that both partners are fully on board with the idea of parenting, as any ambivalence will put a dampener on your sex life.
- Depression can curb your sex drive and confidence, and some of the medications prescribed for depression can decrease libido.[52] It is important to treat the depression first and then address any lasting effects on your sex life.
- Stress and exhaustion can leave you feeling very much not in the mood and may affect sexual function.[53] Your workload might be overwhelming, you might find you just can't say 'no' to your boss, you may have financial pressures building up, or as a classic overachiever you may find you are your own worst enemy.
- Obsessing about Project Baby can make you overly focused on having sex around ovulation, so that you may have forgotten how to have spontaneous sex. Try not to 'go through the motions' as you put baby-making above desire – babies come from love, passion and desire.
- Drinking too much alcohol can reduce sex drive.
- Premature ejaculation or impotence issues for men and painful sex or vaginismus (where the muscles around the vagina involuntarily tense before penetration) will affect your sex life. Do talk to your GP or a counsellor if you are having problems of this kind.
- It is also worth getting your thyroid checked, as this can affect libido.

HOW TO GET SEX BACK ON TRACK

Do:
- Have sex throughout the month, not just at your most fertile times. Regular ejaculation is thought to produce fresher sperm,

which is better than saving it all up for the fertile time of the month when the sperm will have been hanging around the rest of the month in the testicles and may not be the best of the bunch.

- Be discreet about your period and fertile time: you are in this together, but it does not mean you need to share every detail with him. You need to be gently aware of your fertile times, not overly fixated.
- Orgasm for a woman as well as the man is important (although research suggests it is not essential). In a woman it propels the sperm further up into the cervix, which can be quite tricky to pass. In a man it ejaculates sperm from further back in the testicles, where the sperm is fresher and more recently manufactured.
- Maintain an element of surprise; spontaneity is very sexy. Try having sex in different places, not just the bedroom.
- Foreplay is important: it gets the pheromones up and running and makes everything more enjoyable (apparently the pheromones in male perspiration have been shown to reduce a woman's tension and alter the hormone response that regulates the menstrual cycle).[54] Massage and nipple stimulation are enjoyable and help with arousal and relaxation.
- Remember that an important part of sex is the emotional connection you have with the other person; babies are born out of love – love and passion are the vital ingredients. Enjoy sex that is not focused on outcome but is about being in and enjoying the moment. Invest time and attention in your relationship and make love-making a priority. Rediscover your partner as he is now, rather than who he was or who you want him to be.
- Be playful and joyful – it's contagious. If there is something that you need or want, then be the first to give it. Demonstration is the first law of attraction.
- Ideally lie down afterwards, but don't stop yourself urinating, as this can lead to infection.
- Seek professional help if you really feel you can't get your sex life back on track.

Don't:

- Pressurize your partner to perform only at the 'right time of the month' – men need women to want to have sex with them for them, not just to make a baby. I have seen so many times how timing sex to try and conceive can damage a relationship and ultimately not result in a pregnancy. There is nothing less attractive for a man than being used as a baby-making machine. It's important that your partner feels you want to have sex with him because he's the hottest thing on two legs!

- Use lubricants or saliva, as they are hostile to sperm (although there are now specific lubricants available that address this – make sure you read the label).
- Let him know when the ovulation monitor has a smiley face – keep a bit of mystery about your sex life.
- Let your sex life suffer because of overwork. Many couples now work very long hours and are tired and depleted. The knock-on effect is that they suffer from a lack of libido. Add to that the pressure to perform, and it is not hard to see how this can quickly become an issue for couples.
- Become so obsessed with diet and lifestyle issues that you take all the joy out of your life and kill your libido. Don't forget that diet might make a difference, but sex definitely does.

Note: In cases of blocked tubes, poor semen quality and in some other instances, having sex more often will not make a difference, and patients will need to look into assisted reproduction (see pages 206–34).

DOES GOOD SEX INCREASE THE CHANCE OF CONCEPTION?

I certainly believe that the emotional and physical quality of sex, and the time spent thinking and preparing for sex, enhances arousal and fertility. A high level of arousal in men is thought to be associated with better-quality sperm; on the other hand, if the man feels under pressure to produce sperm, performance anxiety can set in. As arousal in women increases, more vaginal lubrication is produced, which is naturally protective for sperm (unless there are pH level issues; see page 174). And the more pleasurable the sex, the more likely you are to have sex more frequently, which of course increases the chances of conception!

It isn't yet known how much female orgasm contributes to conception. Sperm needs about five hours to ripen once it comes into contact with the cervical mucus. Once it has ripened, if orgasm takes place, it can help to move the sperm through the cervix and nearer to its target of the egg, so good sex might help the chances of conception, but the main thing is not to feel pressured.

Good sex is very bonding, so even for same-sex couples who are going through donor insemination or IVF, it's an important part of the process. It's also very enjoyable – much more healthy as a stimulant that most of the things we reach for – plus it's a great relaxant.

In terms of sexual positions, the missionary position is probably best as it allows for deep penetration towards the cervix.

CHINESE MEDICINE AND LIBIDO

Low libido is usually considered to be a weakness in the Kidney energy system, although at my clinic I see an increasing amount of women and men who suffer from Liver Qi Stagnation. This problem arises when there is too much pressure around sex and when there are emotional problems within the relationship. I think this can be linked to couples trying to time sex too precisely and therefore it can become rather forced and tense. With this scenario women are likely to develop ovulation problems, or men may suffer from performance anxiety. Therapies such as massage and acupuncture are very useful to help couples relax. There is nothing worse than being told you just need to 'relax more', but there is a grain of truth in it: tension and sex are not happy bed partners.

The Chinese have a well-documented history of recognizing and treating problems with libido. Many Chinese herbs and formulas for this problem existed long before Viagra. Women's libido needs to be considered as more than just her sexual appetite. In women it is as much to do with your vitality, your self-esteem and the way you feel about your partner. That is not to say sexual appetite is not important; just that women require a different approach to treatment when considering improving their libido. Women require nourishing over a long period of time to slowly and gently build their vitality and reserves so that they regain that loving feeling. It is very different for men, who can perform perfectly well with a short burst of energy; this is why Viagra works – it's a bit like rocket fuel. So for the practitioner of Chinese medicine, when considering acupuncture and herbal medicine, it is important to work very differently with men and women.

Natural libido-boosting toolkit
Foods
- oysters
- watermelon
- chocolate
- asparagus
- avocados
- pumpkin seeds
- celery
- chilli
- figs
- garlic

Herbs
- Ginkgo biloba
- Ginseng
- Horny goat weed
- Maca
- Damiana

Libido and lifestyle
- Alcohol is a depressant. Although one drink can help you relax and enjoy a lovely dinner, finishing off a bottle or two won't be very helpful to your libido.
- Smoking restricts blood flow (essential for sex). For this reason as well as so many others, it's a very good idea to kick the habit.

- Recreational drugs may seem to increase libido temporarily, but they can have a very detrimental effect in the long run.
- Keep fit to improve Blood flow and also self-esteem. Feeling confident is a potent libido booster.

Use your senses

Around ovulation we suddenly find men a lot more attractive than usual and we also seem to attract more attention ourselves. This is all down to pheromones. Research into human mating has found that the effect of scent on males and on females differs. It's thought that men tend to subconsciously notice fertility signals in women, while women notice particularly favourable traits in men that they wouldn't mind passing on to their children. All of these signals are apparently detected through scent. The scent of a man, especially from his armpits, has a powerful effect on female mood and hormones and can increase fertility, so try not to over-sanitize.

And where would love be without food? A delicious meal can be the perfect aphrodisiac and get our senses heightened. It might be a cliché, but when you look at oysters and figs it makes perfect sense why they are two of the most sensual foods. Putting aside a little time for you and your partner and making sure you get to have romantic dates is all part of the baby-making process in my eyes. It's something that often gets forgotten in this hectic world.

Finally, massage is a wonderful way to encourage intimacy: energy flows through loving touch, which can be relaxing and stimulating at the same time. Body specialist Monika Skrzydlewska says that even in these highly sexual times we often overlook our most sensual organ of all, the skin; we need human touch literally to survive and especially to thrive. Even if you haven't had a great deal of practice, simple massage techniques can have a very good effect.

CHAPTER SEVEN
FERTILITY MINDFULNESS

To live long people should take care not to worry too much, not to get too angry, not to get too sad, not to get too frightened, not to do too much, talk too much or laugh too much.

Sun Simiao

Throughout our lives we will experience times of intense emotional difficulty and sometimes unimaginable stress. This is part of the human condition, and in many ways how we cope and adapt to these times will shape us for years to come. For some people, the journey towards becoming a parent can present many challenges and we all respond differently to these. Some people are like the river running gently around the rocks, whereas others will get stuck trying to clamber over them.

Part of my role is to help women through the difficult and often all-consuming emotions they can experience while trying to conceive or going through fertility treatment. Women seem instinctively aware that their emotions can impact on their fertility. Sometimes they will say to me things like: 'I'm stressed that I am stressed, because I know it's bad for me!'

I have felt that for the last ten years, public health messages have been very much focused on good diet, and this has led to many people improving their eating habits and valuing the importance of a healthy diet and beneficial supplements. Of course this is a good thing – a great thing. However, I feel the next area of interest will be the mind and how it is central to our health and wellbeing. Certainly patients are becoming more aware that physical problems can have their roots in emotional difficulties, or that emotional difficulties impact on their physical problems. The mind and the body are not separate.

Patients come to see me with many anxieties and stresses; there is fear of failure, sometimes even a feeling of panic. Some of the patients I see are impatient, and some are busy accumulating more information than they could ever absorb. As humans, we can be competitive and used to getting what we want in life when we want it, and become frustrated when things don't go to plan. Some of us like to have a schedule and have control over our lives, whereas others may need to develop some order and organization. Many are unhappy and experiencing acute feelings of grief and sadness. All of these things can impact on our relationships and our overall sense of wellbeing and, yes, our fertility.

HOW DO YOU KNOW IF YOU'RE STRESSED OUT?

You will tend to know instinctively if stress is getting the better of you, but here are some of the key indicators that remind us when we need to take it easier in life:

- constant tiredness
- avoiding getting things done
- tension, especially in the neck and shoulders
- struggling to sleep well through the night
- loss of appetite or reaching for comfort foods all the time
- feeling distracted and unfocused, perhaps struggling with self-confidence
- a sense of panic about everything you need to get done
- feeling under more pressure than you can cope with
- sighing often
- disrupted digestion
- feeling irritable, defensive or tearful
- overthinking things
- disrupted menstrual cycle

What I want you to develop is a sense of calm and clarity; to be relaxed yet disciplined and to take positive actions without being fixated or obsessed. Learn when to take charge and when to let go. I have huge sympathy for women and couples struggling to conceive, but I have also seen how patients' emotional responses can become part of the problem. It is important to find peace within ourselves; we can learn so much when we realize that some of the stresses in our lives are generated from within, and that we have the power to choose how we react to what life brings us. I am not saying you are to blame for anything, only that you have within you the power to make things easier – more simple.

I want to teach you how to cultivate emotional wellness and to learn how to identify some of the stresses that you might be creating or contributing to. Identifying the areas we can work on in our lives and understanding how we ourselves can be mindful can have far-reaching benefits. We can be mindful about our menstrual cycle, being aware of our body as it changes throughout the month. We can eat mindfully, which has been shown to improve the digestion and absorption of food. We can develop an awareness about how we create stress for ourselves and how we can change this pattern. And of course we can be mindful with our partners – I probably should have put that first.

OUR EMOTIONAL STRENGTHS, OUR EMOTIONAL WEAKNESSES

When I first meet a patient I always think to myself: 'Who is this person and what makes them tick?' I want to connect with my patients at a deep level and to be able to understand the source of their imbalances. What are the stresses in their lives? The clues are usually there in something they say or the way they say it, or the way they hold themselves as they describe their fertility journey to this point of coming along to see me. I have discovered over years of experience that while we are all a mix of many different emotions, we do tend towards a particular type, our true nature, which is both our main strength and our main weakness or vulnerability.

I hope as I describe the following emotional tendencies you will recognize how the body and mind interact. My aim is that you should develop your own awareness and toolkit for when things feel out of balance. I have outlined five personality types, and you will no doubt identify more strongly with one of these. This is your true nature, but around that nature the other four types will coexist. So if you identify more strongly with one type, that does not mean you do not possess elements of all of them, just that your innate strengths and weaknesses are more profoundly explained by one. Perhaps you will recognize yourself as the over-thinking type with a tendency to digestive problems. Or maybe the excited, enthusiastic, fluttery Heart type, who can be so strong but then suddenly feel a lack of joy and in danger of burning out. See which of these characters speaks to you the most, and if you ever feel your strength turning into a weakness, try some of the methods I have suggested for your type. This will enable you to make better choices about what helps you and what tends to make things worse. As you feel more connected to your true nature, you will feel a great sense of connection to your life and those around you. In this way you will become more balanced and fertile as you try for a baby.

All Heart

'I'll put my heart and soul into this and then I'll know I will have done everything in my power to have a baby.'

Those of you who are ruled by your hearts have many things to be thankful for. All Heart types are engaged, excited and enthusiastic about life. They have great drive and give their all – to relationships, to new projects, to everything. They will take risks, which can lead to great growth. They are filled with optimism; they love attention, give attention, are very emotionally intelligent, loyal, empathetic and their passion is infectious, as is their laughter, which sometimes bursts out extra loudly and not always at quite the right time. They wear their heart on their sleeve. Heart types are able to laugh things off, making little of their pain and hardship. They will communicate all of it to you, every last detail in an honest and upfront manner. But then so as not to burden you with the suffering of it they will add a throwaway comment like 'There are millions of people worse off than me', or make a joke at their own expense. Such is the generosity of the Heart type.

Heart types will often have bright eyes, soft skin and a warm energy. They are able to turn the mundane into the extraordinary. They are often intuitive and persuasive, generous in spirit and passionate about the pleasures life has to offer.

When things don't go so well, the Heart type can give so much that she tips from enthusiasm and excitement into feeling a lack in some way – often a lack of joy, such an empty feeling when you are all heart. Heart types can be fragile: they shine so bright that sometimes they can feel as though they will burn out. They can suddenly feel anxious that if they are not fabulous then somehow they are a burden. Excitement can transform into feeling agitated, hyped up and wired, making it difficult to sleep or relax. Think of Tigger in *Winnie-the-Pooh*. Bouncing, bouncing, bouncing, full of the joys, and then . . . disaster. The highs and the lows. Warmth may turn to melancholy; there is a feeling of restlessness, perhaps a sense of dread or panic, and they can feel nervous and unfocused. Boundaries blur and they begin to crave the wrong kinds of stimulation, as passion turns into hedonism and enthusiasm into compulsion.

When it comes to fertility, Heart types are often blessed with something called the 'optimism bias'.[55] Studies have shown that generally people who are more optimistic are more successful, even lucky. The flip side is that occasionally too much optimism means too much risk-taking with one's health. The confident 'I'll be OK' can become a vulnerability at the last moment, feeling suddenly afraid to hope after giving so much. Heart types can be prone to circulatory problems, anxiety and even palpitations or panic attacks. They might have a lined forehead, and they may need to look after their nervous system. The Heart person loves to love and craves it in return. They just need to be aware of maintaining a balance, as there is a tendency not always to listen to others.

In IVF, these patients give their all and are really focused and optimistic. One lovely All Heart patient of mine announced as she began her IVF cycle, 'I really rather like IVF: it's like *George's Marvellous Medicine* mixing up all the baby-making drugs.'

However, if someone says something to knock this positivity, they can suddenly crash. Often they will wobble after embryo collection; having held it together the entire way through with boundless energy and optimism, suddenly the self-doubt can creep in. When their positivity turns to negativity, they torture themselves with morbid thoughts and can become withdrawn and full of dread.

Toolbox

- You need to learn to balance your lovely exuberant nature with solitude and calm.
- Give yourself plenty of space and time and don't feel rushed.
- Consider couples counselling if things become strained, and make time to get together properly with your partner for non-fertility-related activities.
- Learning to conserve your energy is key for you, because you easily give your energy away as you are so good at communicating and connecting with everyone around you.
- Borrow a friend's child and take them out or have a cuddle.
- Connect with the people you love: confide in someone and open your heart to them.
- Learn to keep just a little bit back.
- Learn to withdraw, but don't cut yourself off in the process; you don't have to be all or nothing.
- Relaxation is essential for Heart types so that they can calm and regenerate that amazing energy they have.
- Definitely do yoga.
- Meditation is a really good idea. When you meditate, focus on helping your body to cool down through cooling thoughts. Prayers of any kind and rituals are good for the Heart.
- Make your surroundings vibrant: light candles and wrap up warm in front of the fire.
- Massage with rose oil.
- Hold something back for yourself. Don't always be the one to engage in everything, or volunteer to do more than you can. Learn how to say 'no'.
- You can easily become overheated and dehydrated, so make sure you drink plenty of water and are properly hydrated at all times.
- Avoid heating and drying foods like curry, sugar, alcohol, coffee, tea and salt. Eat plenty of alfalfa, rye, asparagus and papaya.
- Tea: rosebud.

My personal meditation is more powerful if I can also meditate upon others who are trying to start a family.

Kaf Lamed Yud (Hebrew)

FERTILITY AS CREATIVITY

'The greatest unconscious force in the lives of children is the unfulfilled dreams of their parents.'

Carl Jung

Conceiving a baby is the most creative act we as humans are capable of: conception is quite literally the creation of life. I believe it is really important to have passion and purpose in life, and I see many women reach a time in their life when they feel they are lacking something. For the women I see in my clinic it is a baby they yearn for; often they will have the job, the house and the husband, but despite all of that they feel they are missing something. I often advise women who are feeling this lack of joy and passion to engage in something else that honours their creativity. Allowing themselves to have joy and purpose in life is an important aspect of their fertility. I have seen many, many times that when a woman gently shifts her focus to her own needs, she then conceives her longed-for child. In Chinese medicine we see a strong connection between the Heart and the Womb. What nourishes the Heart nourishes the Womb.

The Thinker

'I'm fine!'

The Thinker has many great strengths. Thinkers are able to fend for themselves very well and have a capacity for high self-esteem, optimism and great fairness. They are open to receiving as well as giving nourishment on all levels. When everything is in balance, their thought process is clear and they are also very caring towards other people. The Thinker is attentive, a good peacemaker, skilled at connecting with people and putting them at ease, chameleon-like, always able to set the space and mood for others. They are grounded and often quite serene or poised when balanced, able to alter their perspective and see things from all sides, although more sympathetic than empathetic. Even the Thinker's body will be naturally curved. She facilitates action, is easy and relaxed.

When things go a little haywire, though, Thinkers will tend to start overthinking, analysing everything to the nth degree. Perhaps a trigger questions the Thinker's sense of self-worth, self-love, and so she begins to worry, to become more muddled and less able to act or make decisions. She might go round and round the houses, procrastinating, not sure what to do next. I even know of overthinkers who struggle to get their sentences out when feeling under pressure or stuck in their thoughts. And the trouble is that if unaware of this, the Thinker will often be very slow to ask for or to accept help, declaring 'I'm fine' to anyone who asks. The positive ability to fend for themselves turns into self-absorption and overcompensation. They will start to look inwards rather than outwards; they may become less sympathetic, apathetic, defeated, tangled up in details and feel saturated to the point of inertia. Self-confidence can turn into self-pity, churning things over, procrastinating rather than taking action or decisions. In this state the Thinker is no longer able to digest information so well or make it useful, and she might lose her usual sense of natural and healthy boundaries, both in her lifestyle and relationships.

The organ associated with the Thinker is the stomach – our ability to absorb. Scientists now think of the stomach as the body's 'second brain': there are so many nerve endings there and it is so sensitive to the mind. So once you start thinking too much and struggle to process those thoughts, the stomach similarly begins to struggle with the digestion process. Often stools become loose or lurch from loose to overly hard or constipated on some days. When in balance, though, the Thinker has a very healthy appetite and keeps their weight at a natural happy medium. Plus their skin is nicely toned. Out of balance, they often tend to put on weight more easily, crave sugar or starch and the skin might become a little flabby, too yielding.

With fertility, over-thinking can lead easily to obsession and a heightened state of worry, which doesn't make for a very receptive environment. The key is to remind yourself to look outwards, to let go, to start doing more things that come naturally, to follow that brilliant gut of yours. I see so many patients who go into information overload when it comes to fertility, accumulating knowledge for the sake of it rather than taking action. For these patients, the quest for a baby can become an obsession, taking over their every thought, but they are so weighed down with thought they become unable to act.

During IVF, the Thinker will become very focused on the minutiae. They will know the exact size of each follicle and the exact thickness of the endometrium and they will be hungry for every bit of information. But all of this information only adds to the anxiety; it is important to develop a sense of trust in the process, as you can easily become despondent when things aren't going to plan.

Toolbox

- It's important to recognize your own needs and to learn to express these needs. Part of your habit of collecting information is because you are quietly trying to take care of things internally so as not to be a burden on others. But a problem shared is a problem halved, so learning to be more demonstrative will help you no end. So next time you are about to say 'I'm fine', stop for a moment and ask yourself if the person asking how you are might be able to do anything to support you.
- Do something for yourself every day.
- Learning to ask for help is key for you. Your natural inclination is to want to support others, but you easily feel unsupported yourself when your needs are not met; so be honest about this. When we do things for others, we are often fulfilling a need within ourselves, which is fine, but you need to balance this with knowing what your needs are and getting them met too.
- Avoid long monologues about yourself; instead, tell someone one thing you need every day.
- Overthinkers need to have some boundaries of the mind, not in a rigid way, but to give yourself back a sense of regularity.
- Feel the fear and do it anyway.
- The Thinker benefits a great deal from human touch, so a massage can do wonders, especially from the one who loves you.
- You have a tendency to accumulate 'stuff', be it emotional or belongings. Declutter your house and try to change your ways, to let go more.
- Regular eating is very good for the Thinker. They will often be people who get moody when their blood sugar drops and they haven't eaten for a few hours.

- Be at one with nature and feel the earth beneath your feet. A walk will clear the head and get things moving if you are feeling stuck, whether in body or mind.
- Eat plenty of digestion-supporting foods: sweet vegetables like squash and carrots, plus grains such as oats and quinoa, aromatic herbs and spices like basil, ginger and cinnamon, as well as green tea, fennel and rocket.
- Don't eat things straight out of the fridge.
- Eat little but often, and keep meals light in the evenings so as not to overload the digestion.
- Train yourself to replace the question 'What's wrong with me?' with a positive focus on the next thing you need to do. Repeat to yourself positive statements like: 'I am well nourished in all areas of my life and I have everything I need.'
- The part of this book that will help you the most is the In the Fertility Kitchen, but be careful not to obsess about food.
- Tea: aniseed or cardamom.

LISTENING TO THE PAIN

I have learnt both through my work and as a yoga student that there is a gift that comes from pure focus: the gift of simplicity. I have also learnt that we cannot hide from pain, because it is from pain that transformation can occur. Pain indicates where we have the most to learn and grow. I was reminded on a yoga course that some postures are effortless and make us feel good and in the flow, but in other postures we feel deep discomfort and our natural reaction is to want to move away from that. Yoga teaches us to gently go to those places of tension and discomfort because those are the areas that need our attention the most. The more we are able to work on those areas, the easier and more simple things become.

The Perfectionist

'I feel like a failure; everything is in its place except the baby.'

The Perfectionist seeks beauty; they are discerning, keepers of standards and have an ability to create order from chaos. For the Perfectionist, everything has its place. They often love creativity but will also be brilliant with schedules, unflappable in most situations and appreciated (if not lauded) for their consistency, integrity, their methodical ways and accepting natures. They are neither gullible nor easily upset; they are an island of calm. Perfectionists are highly principled. Everything in life has a place and is well organized. They know the order of things; and if you go about things in the right way then the rule is everything should follow at the right time, just as it's meant to. Everything has a system, a place, a meaning, a role.

These types strive for perfection, but striving sometimes leads to disappointment when the world doesn't fit their sense of how things should be. When feeling under pressure or out of balance, the Perfectionist might begin to over-identify with her strong principles, so that she seems unwilling to let go of control. In the strive for perfection lies the potential for disappointment, which can lead to the Perfectionist falling back on safe ground, rituals, habits and old patterns of thinking. Their usual unflappable self may become sloppy and a tendency towards self-righteousness can creep in. Others may find it hard to meet the Perfectionist's exacting standards. Often there are suppressed emotions at play: an old grief, disappointment or hurt that hasn't been expressed and let go. As Perfectionists detest confrontation, there may be old disagreements lurking, or a sadness about settling and accepting perhaps a little too much, rather than grasping the beauty and spontaneity in their character and in life.

In the body, these suppressed emotions will often sit in the lungs. It might feel as though it is hard to breathe deeply and freely. This also affects the intestines, leading to constipation. The body becomes as stuck as the mind and emotions.

The fertility journey can be hard for those who seek perfection. They will be the ones who are precisely timing sex and doing everything by the proverbial book. They will methodically alter their diets, their sex lives, their social lives, their alcohol intake; every detail of their lives will be managed, measured and recorded. There will be a tendency to minimize setbacks with a stalwart 'Oh, it's no big deal, really.' But underneath there may be a danger of real disappointment and they might forget to enjoy the journey.

The IVF process itself won't be an issue; it will probably appeal to their exacting nature with its precise measurements and timings. The discipline won't pose a problem, and as long as it all goes to plan, they will cope quite well. Faith in the professionals will be key: it will be important that they feel the clinic knows what they are doing and can live up to their high standards. For example, they won't like it if someone hasn't read their notes or fully informed themselves about their case. The Perfectionist will find it difficult to trust, but as long as they sense things are well organized and the professionals are on the ball, they will feel OK.

Toolbox

- Breathing exercises are a very effective way for getting the energy gently moving again and unblocking emotions (see page 183). Walk outdoors in the countryside if possible to breathe the air.
- With all my fertility patients, I encourage them to let go of past hurts wherever possible, so that they can once again feel that lightness and gentle excitement of possibility, of the new, of the unexpected. Consider counselling if you find this particularly difficult (see Resources).
- Skin brushing helps the lymphatic system to move energy around the body and encourages the skin to breathe; the skin is often described as the 'second lung'.
- If you are experiencing an inability to let go and it affects your digestion (you may experience constipation, for example), then colonic irrigation may be a good idea.
- Clear out the clutter in your life. Go through your cupboards and give everything a spring clean. If you haven't worn something for a year, give it to charity. Make space for the new.
- If you have past hurts that you are struggling to let go of, try writing a letter of angst followed by a letter of thanks (see page 141). If your hurts or disappointments stem from childhood, don't be afraid to write a letter of angst to your parents – not to send, but to allow yourself to truly express the hurt. Pour out your feelings. And then write about what you are thankful for in your life today: the people, the moments – all the little details.

- Some Perfectionists may have old issues with the father–daughter relationship, perhaps seeking a father figure or idealizing one's father. You might wish to explore these issues in therapy.
- Remember the times in your life when crises turned into opportunities, when you found the silver lining. Become an alchemist: turn negative into positive and the glass will become half full, which is just how the Perfectionist likes it. An appreciation diary is very helpful, as is telling loved ones what you appreciate about them and also acknowledging your own achievements.
- Nurture your creativity with a 'mood board' (see page 139) and bring beauty into your life at every turn.
- Write a letter to an old or lost loved one, or even to your younger self. Read it aloud and then burn it or let it fly away in the wind. Embrace any tears that flow with the release.
- Tea: sage or ginger.

The Visionary

'I'm afraid that I will never be pregnant.'

The Visionary is relentless in their quest for the truth. Some would call them philosophers: they scrutinize life, ever watchful, curious, always seeking. A Visionary has an uncanny ability to uncover things, and they will feel a strong connection to their 'destiny'. They are often articulate but in a self-contained way, even enigmatic. They are detailed, imaginative, curious but careful, always honest, usually very modest and fascinated with life. When in good balance, knowledge combines with wisdom and power with compassion. They see right into the heart of the matter. Resilient by nature, they are born survivors who can bounce back from many knock-backs; they are tough with deep reserves of strength – emotionally, the Visionary is a rock.

The problem with rocks is that they can be quite hard; they can literally become frozen with fear. When under excess pressure, the Visionary will begin to experience more of a fear of failure. Their confidence and courage may begin to drain away as their energy reserves deplete and they work too hard. They can become negative and cynical and sabotage their own happiness by making things harder than they need to be. They can become withdrawn; insight turns into sarcasm and observation into criticism. Strong visionary skills can lead to seeing the worst in situations and imagining bleak outcomes. They might become overly fussy or isolated and retreat from life. Always candid, they can become tactless. They can tend towards hypochondria, a combination of their imagination and fears. At their worst, the Visionary can become a bit of a moaner, I'm afraid.

The fears associated with fertility can especially drain the Visionary's sexual energy and libido, and so fear feeds itself, as having sex less frequently makes conception less likely. Often anxiety manifests itself in the body through lower back pain or urinary problems. Ear problems are common among Visionary types.

The fertility journey can be quite hard for the Visionary, because they will want to get to the truth and the reasons for whatever is happening in their body. Sometimes such truths are hard to come by, and when concrete reasons are not provided, the Visionary may tend to turn quite cynical, suffer from a loss of hope and become defeatist. On the positive side, if Visionaries can stay balanced, their wonderfully resilient nature keeps them determined to conceive and this special willpower stands them in good stead.

During IVF treatment, the Visionary might find herself wanting to retreat and cut herself off. She might find it hard if the reasons behind the fertility problem are less than 100 per cent clear, because she will want to understand those reasons and the wisdom in going ahead with an IVF plan. Without a clear way ahead the Visionary can feel a little lost, but I always encourage these patients to keep the faith and stay connected because they have such strong resources and a stronger will than most. It's good for them to keep asking questions and double-checking advice, as seeking the truth is where they feel most comfortable.

Toolbox

- Don't be afraid to go slow. The key is to find the balance between doing and resting that is right for you and your body. Get to know the level of activity and work that energizes you, and where it tips over into beginning to deplete your reserves. If your fears ever become so great that you feel at all overwhelmed, counselling is always an excellent thing to consider. It is OK to take some of the weight and responsibility from your shoulders.
- Keep a strong vision of what you are trying to achieve and keep the faith.

- Draw on those deep reserves of steely strength you possess, and connect with the energy of the generations of women in your family who have done this before you. Let them be your strength.
- As well as being strong, work on being tender and open too – try to develop a softer approach. Softness is not weakness; instead see it as a counterbalance to your strong will and sense of self-possession.
- Remember that conception is a receptive act: you must learn to soften and yield as well as defend and protect.
- Try to connect more to others and not cut yourself off emotionally. For example, exercising in a class with other people rather than by yourself is a good idea.
- Try to understand your energy better; don't overexercise and be aware of when you are tired.
- With more rest, your energy reserves will build and courage will come again, as this is your great strength. Try some relaxation or breathing exercises (see page 183) and incorporate some gentle exercise into your day that is relaxing but also gets your energy flowing. Walking is the simplest form of exercise and one of the best.
- Keep a dream diary to help develop your Visionary skills.
- Rest and warmth will build up your reserves; try a lovely heat-wrap treatment and acupuncture with hot needles to warm your body and drive out Coldness. Take a relaxing bath.
- One of my favourite books is *The Compassionate Mind* by Paul Gilbert (see Resources). He describes an exercise in which the object is to limit your criticism of others, because those who are critical of others are actually very critical of themselves. In the exercise you try to limit your criticism of others and yourself, monitor yourself and just observe, then ask why you were critical and what the source of fear is in you. When critical of others this often comes from a feeling of inadequacy within ourselves or from a feeling of fear. So instead of always outwardly projecting these uncomfortable feelings onto another it is more helpful to examine our own nature and attend to our own needs. This is how we will grow and develop spiritually and emotionally. And most of all, practise compassion to yourself and others.
- Eat plenty of seaweed and sushi. Stay in and make soup.
- Tea: jasmine.

IF A FACE CAN TELL A THOUSAND STORIES

'Some people, no matter how old they get, never lose their beauty, they merely move it from their face into their heart.'

Martin Buxbaum

Face diagnosis is part of how I pick up clues about a patient's imbalances or emotional tendencies. The state of the skin, its colouring and tone – all these give me vital clues, which when put together with the patient's other symptoms begin to tell a story.

For me, the biggest indicators of fertility on the face are the philtrum and the ear. The philtrum is the fleshy channel between the nose and above the centre of the top lip. It should be pink and plump. If it is very pale, this tells me that this woman is too Cold, perhaps with a Cold uterus. This can be confirmed by touching the stomach and also the inside of the lower leg between the ankle and knee. If these areas are cold to the touch, I advise the patient to increase warming foods, and I will also apply treatments to add more warmth to the body. I am often able to assess the improvement in the patient's fertility over the course of time by seeing the improvement in the philtrum.

Large, fleshy ear lobes have long been associated with strong constitution or strong Jing. The larger and fleshier the lobe, the stronger the person's inherited constitution is thought to be.

Frustration and impatience is also easy to see on the face: these feelings tend to result in deep frown lines between the eyebrows. A line coming down the face from the outside corner of the eye through the cheek denotes sadness and grief. A line down the face from the corner of the inside of the eye indicates a broken heart or love disappointment.

The tip of the nose tells me about the Heart and how strong the Blood and circulation are, while the mouth and lips tell me about the digestion: a large mouth indicates strong digestion.

The eyes are thought to be the window to our soul, and they relate to the Liver. Often when our vision for life is thwarted, our eyes will be affected in some way.

The Planner

'I'm frustrated because I always planned to have a baby by now.'

The Planner has such a clear vision of life. Every last detail is scheduled, and they are brilliantly organized. If you need a good strategy, ask a Planner. They work hard to succeed, are committed, always well prepared and love a challenge. Planners are active, great doers, with bags of energy. They have a strong sense of independence, curiosity and innovative vision, always going where others might be a little more fearful to tread. For Planners, the solution to any problems will tend to be – you guessed it! – a plan. When they are in balance, they embrace growth and change. There is great strength in a Planner, and at their best they are like a tree bending in the wind: stable and yet yielding at the same time – strength with softness.

When out of balance, the Planner can feel frustrated. They work so hard to make sure everything goes to plan, but life doesn't always have the same thing in mind. When plans are thwarted, they may experience outbursts of anger; their body may become tight, their voice clipped, they'll seem always on alert. Emotionally they can become rigid, no longer being able to see the wood for the trees. That natural feeling of invincible strength becomes a vulnerability and a fear of losing control, which in turn can lead to aggression, loss of perspective and confrontation. The Planner makes the rules, but then feels an urge to break them. They might become extreme, and extremely inconsistent, perhaps on a health kick one day and drinking everyone under the table the next. When tired, strengths turn into weaknesses, and the Planner can become indecisive and scatterbrained, irritable and easily frustrated or angered. Confidence in their goals turns into a feeling of deflation, and their sleep pattern may become irregular as pressure builds up. The organ associated with the Planner is the liver: it is our powerhouse and the organ of action. But in order to act effectively, we need to be both well prepared and prepared to be spontaneous and flexible.

When I meet patients who tend towards planning and therefore frustration, I always notice that they ask me outright for a clear plan they can follow: a diet plan, a relaxation plan, a sex plan! If they are happily in balance, plans can be effective, but if they have become too attached to planning everything in infinite detail, often the best thing I can do is give them nothing faintly resembling a plan and instead ask them to trust me and go with the flow. This isn't to take away their amazing sense of vision, but rather to add a sense of adaptability, to become more of a free and easy wanderer. It is so frustrating for the Planner to find themselves at the mercy of nature, to realize that sometimes working hard enough isn't the answer to being able to conceive.

Planners cope quite well mentally with IVF because there is a plan in place and they can follow it. They are focused and ready to achieve their outcome – a baby. The problems arise for them when things don't go according to plan and they have no control. They also find the two-week wait to find out whether the embryo has implanted very demanding. Without a clear task, they can feel a loss of control. They won't want to take it easy during this time; they will want to fill every waking hour with activity and things to do and achieve, afraid of being alone with their thoughts.

Physically the Planner is strong when in balance, but can tend towards tightness and tension when feeling out of sorts. They may sigh frequently in frustration and might suffer from irregularities in their menstrual cycle and sleep patterns. You may have a tendency to become bloated and can suffer from swollen breasts and abdomen. This can happen during the menstrual cycle but also through an IVF cycle. Bloodshot, watery or slightly yellow eyes are a sign of being out of balance for the Planner, and frown lines may also become pronounced.

Toolbox

- Make a plan, a realistic plan, and set out how you will achieve it. Make it pleasing and enjoyable. Choose for it to be easy.
- You are happiest when things are kept moving. Qi Gong is an excellent exercise for Planners. It encourages a lovely flow of energy around the body, balancing things out (see page 107).
- Yoga stretches will help to release any build-up of tension in the body. Flexibility and flow are a wonderful tonic for the Planner.
- Try to see things from others' points of view. Try saying to them, 'I think you may be feeling . . .'

- Take time out to reflect and contemplate, instead of always forging forward.
- Your shoulders and the base of the skull can get very stiff, so neck and shoulder massages are beneficial. This also helps relieve tension headaches.
- Planners will often suffer from PMS, and then feel much better after their period. See page 182 for tips on managing PMS.
- Learn to balance work with leisure, because your natural inclination is only to stop when exhausted.
- Avoid alcohol and fatty foods and look after your liver. Consider a gentle colonic (see Appendix I).
- Eat more apples, lemons, limes, olives and berries.
- Learn to stay flexible, both emotionally and physically.
- Teas: fennel, nettle.

HOW DIFFERENT EMOTIONS AFFECT US

For each of the five types there is an emotion that will tend to affect us more strongly when we are out of balance, as indicated in the brackets.

- FEAR (Visionary): Diminishes energy and our drive for life. Takes away our will to cope and to survive.
- ANGER (Planner): Blocks our vision for life and makes us frustrated and irritable. Causes us to lash out at life.
- WORRY (Thinker): Makes us anxious and needy. Leads to ruminating on our problems and self-obsession.
- SHOCK (All Heart): Scatters our energy and weakens us. Leaves us anxious and lacking in confidence.
- GRIEF (Perfectionist): Stops us from engaging in life and keeps us from moving forward. Isolates us and prevents us from letting go.

CHANGING HABITS, CHANGING PATTERNS

We can be very habitual creatures and inflexible when confronted with change. Sometimes we may find that the way we do things isn't working anymore and may even be allowing us to stay stuck in a negative pattern. Sometimes in order to make space for something new to come into our lives, we need to let go of something else – make a sacrifice. I have seen many times that when women make changes, it can bring about deeper changes and sometimes that leads to pregnancy.

Think of it as making space for the baby to come into your life. Some people say to me, 'I'll cut down on my workload once I'm pregnant.' I always reply, 'If you know you are working too hard, why not do it now?'

I don't believe couples should give up everything in their pursuit to have a baby, but it's about shifting priorities. At some point in life, certain things become more important than others. Of course we all need to work to earn a living, but you can still work while prioritizing your health. In the same way, it is possible to change your eating habits without taking away all the pleasure of food and cooking. You can reform your drinking habits, but you can still have a drink from time to time. It's about making adjustments and feeling good about it.

It can be really helpful to take on a positive new habit and get rid of a negative one at the same time. So you might want to give up sugar and take up a bit of exercise. Or stop smoking and take up dancing. Try to just do one thing at a time, so take up one positive and let go of one negative. The only person who can prioritize your health is you. So ask yourself: why not?

My friend went on a course to help her quit smoking, and on the course they made you gradually change all your positive associations with smoking. The idea was to break all the habits that you had formed around smoking, from where you bought your cigarettes to your preferred brand and every activity associated with the habit. So if you liked to smoke while chatting on the phone, you were no longer allowed to do that. If you smoked while drinking alcohol, you couldn't do that anymore. You had to switch to a brand you didn't like or associate with anything positive. You had to smoke the cigarette while holding it in a different way to normal. In the end, you were left facing the corner of the room, smoking a brand you didn't like and if anyone tried to talk you had to say, 'Don't talk to me – I'm smoking.' She said they made you carry on smoking right up until the end of the course, and by the end she was absolutely desperate to stop.

To get started you might want to make a plan and enlist a support person who can encourage you and keep you motivated. Here are some things to help you make lasting changes.

- Make a commitment and tell the people around you about the change you are going to make.
- Find someone to support you – someone positive and who you respect.
- Build rewards into your week.
- Take it one day at a time.
- Talk about your positive new habit, especially to people who are interested in it. So if the change is to your diet, talk to people about recipes and food and engage in the subject in as many positive ways as possible.
- When talking or thinking about the habit you have dropped, try not to see it as having 'given up' something. Try just to think of it as 'changing habits'.
- Just like my friend who gave up smoking, try to disassociate from anything positive about the old habit. The mind can play tricks on you and make you believe it wasn't that bad – even about smoking, which we know is damaging to our health.
- If you fail, reflect on what went wrong and try again, safeguarding against the aspect that made you fail the first time.

Changing habits

When I first trained to be an acupuncturist we had a professor of Chinese medicine who would come over from China to teach us. He was a man of few words, and we mostly just observed how he did things. He did not encourage questions, only observation. This is typical of the difference between the West and the East: in the West we want knowledge very, very quickly; we want to run before we can walk and we want answers to everything. But in the East there is a belief that real knowledge is acquired slowly, through careful observation and many hours of practice. And so we were encouraged to observe.

I noticed that the professor would sometimes change something to do with the patients while they were lying on the couch with their needles in place. He might move their shoes to the other side of the bed, or put their coat in a different place to where they had left it. Although this was done subtly, it was clear to me that it was done quite deliberately. On a couple of occasions he caught my gaze: there was a little twinkle in his eye, as if he was encouraging me to think about what he was doing. Later he asked me: 'So why do you think I am moving these items?' I told him that I felt he was trying to change the way the patient did things; acupuncture, after all, is about changing energy. By moving the patient's belongings, he was reinforcing the need for change, but also allowing them to partake in the change themselves. He nodded wisely without saying a word, but I definitely saw that little twinkle in his eye. Sometimes the best teachers are the ones that say the least and let us work things out for ourselves. I have certainly never forgotten this lesson. Sometimes, however much we resist things, change is inevitable and may just bring you back into balance and make you more fertile.

CHOOSE YOUR WORDS IMPECCABLY (FROM *THE FOUR AGREEMENTS* BY DON MIGUEL RUIZ)

I think we all have a responsibility to choose our words carefully. Words have a resonance, a vibration, and they can really hurt other people. In his book *The Four Agreements*, Don Miguel Ruiz describes words as being like seeds that are sown in the garden of our minds to grow and influence us for years to come.

I learn a great deal about a patient by the language they use: it tells me about how they are feeling and what energy they might be attracting to themselves through their own words. I might hear such things as:

- 'My body is a disaster – it always lets me down!'
- 'I have always known I'd struggle to have a baby.'
- 'This will kill me.'

Equally, sometimes the words that medics use or the sentiment they convey can be negative and damaging. Expressions such as 'incompetent cervix', 'low ovarian reserve' and 'poor responder' may be medically correct, but they can also be tough to hear, especially if you are already feeling vulnerable.

I had a patient who told me that her headmistress had once said of her: 'Some people are put on this earth to work and some people aren't. Sarah is one of those people who was just not made for work!' This is clearly nonsense, and how a grown woman could put such an idea in the head of a fifteen-year-old girl is just wrong in so many ways. Did it affect her? Yes, I think it did. She tended towards overwork and overachieving – clearly her way of trying to prove her old headmistress wrong. It seems crazy that all these years later and having achieved many things in her life she could be proud of, this statement still dented Sarah's self-belief.

It is not just the words of others that affect us; the words that we choose to use can resonate back at us. For instance, if you were to say, 'So-and-so is ugly and rude', what you are doing is making those words reflect back at you. The person you are talking to cannot see the person you are talking about and so those words attach themselves to you and not the absent person. Here are some pointers to bear in mind:

- The words you use will reflect back on you and become a truth about yourself and your fertility.
- Try to avoid negative language or exaggerating needlessly, for example: 'My period pain was horrific!' Horrific is a word to describe terrible atrocities; as painful as periods can be, they are rarely horrific. By using the word, you attract drama to yourself.
- Engage in the sharing of interesting and creative ideas.
- Don't engage in fault-finding and criticism. When you criticize others, you are often really talking about yourself.
- Speak and choose your words from a place of love and compassion.
- Don't be a victim; take responsibility for yourself and don't play the blame game. Don't say: 'Why does this always happen to me!'

- Don't moan – moaning is catching. It's good to talk through emotional difficulties, but moaning is something different!
- Don't gossip; my grandmother taught me that 'only boring people gossip'! Talk about your ideas and inspirations instead.
- Avoid using statements like 'I felt like my insides were being ripped out' – it creates a bad visual image for you and those listening.
- Don't attack with words.
- Don't be always on the defensive. Many people are so focused on being right that they forget being happy is far more important.
- Positive affirmations help us create positive realities. Try repeating to yourself positive mantras, such as 'I am fertile and I have everything I need to have a baby.'
- Use words with a positive vibration – words of quality and integrity.

   'Most folks are about as happy as they make up their minds to be.'

                                                           Abraham Lincoln

MOOD BOARDS

I am not one for lists; in fact, I have been told I am quite bad at responding to lists of instructions. I prefer to find other ways to manifest the things I want in my life. One of the things I like to do is to make a mood board. I am quite a visual person and sometimes doing this helps me straighten my thinking and prioritize.

It can be very therapeutic to collect images and scraps of fabric and words that appeal to you and put them together on a board. Then you can spend some time everyday looking at your board and focusing on bringing that energy into your life. Creative people use this tool all the time: graphic designers use mood boards to enable them to illustrate visually the style or direction they are pursuing.

I think it is best not to think too much about it when you first start, but to be quite free in your thinking. There isn't really a right or a wrong. Observe what you place in the centre of the board – I tend to see this as a central issue, something of importance. I have quite often readjusted the central image after constructing my board, as it might be something I am giving more attention than I need to. Sometimes I find when I shift that image from the central position and replace it with something else, things change.

A patient of mine told me how she had made a mood board and had placed something associated with work at the centre. When she noticed this, she moved a picture of a baby to the centre instead. Now of course it isn't as if she suddenly fell pregnant, but she did remember to reassess her priorities and to focus on the image of a baby. Or it could be the other way around: you might be overly focused on having a baby at the expense of everything else, and there may be other aspects of your life you need to nurture and bring to the centre.

I like to use lots of words on my mood boards, words that have a positive vibration or that relate to areas I need to work on. I remember I put the words 'grace', 'women', 'health' and 'healing' on one board, and three months later I was approached by an old friend and colleague of mine asking me to join a new women's health club called Grace he was involved in. I had a little chuckle to myself – had I manifested this into my life, or was it just a coincidence?

What I do know is that when we focus on the negative, we create tension in our body, and that tension blocks our creativity, making it harder for us to make good choices for ourselves. I am sure looking at positive images and words that have a good vibration helps us to feel better about the world and also to recognize the things that are important to us. This can, in turn, make us more receptive.

I know many couples who, in their struggle to conceive, sometimes forget what it is they are trying to bring into their lives. A gentle visual reminder every day may help.

Letting go of the past: a letter of angst

As we prepare to become parents ourselves, it's a good time to let go of the past, particularly any angst we might be harbouring towards our own parents. This exercise is especially helpful for Perfectionists.

If you are holding on to any hurts or frustrations, this is the time to pour them out. Visualize how you felt growing up: remember any hurts that you had that you have been carrying around with you for many years, or comments or attitudes that have shaped you and become part of what you believe about yourself. Those thoughts and feelings become part of our make-up, part of who we are – or think we are. Some of these beliefs are useful, and some are not; some stay with us for a long time and they can really do us a disservice. So your letter of angst is an opportunity to get these feelings out. By putting them down on paper and acknowledging the hurt you feel, you will be taking the first step towards ridding yourself of these emotions forever.

Here are some cues to get you started:

- 'When you said X to me, it made me feel Y . . .'
- 'When you told me I was X, it made me feel Y . . .'
- 'I am sure you did not mean to hurt me, but when you did X, you really hurt me because it made me feel Y . . .'
- 'I have carried this feeling of X around with me for many years and now I want to be free from it.'

Bear with me here: it might not be immediately apparent that this would have any impact on your fertility per se, but the environmental and emotional climate in which we had our earliest experiences are the foundations upon which we were formed. For better or for worse, these influences shaped us, so it's good to make your peace at this important time in your life and let go of the past while looking to the future.

Write as many letters as you feel you need to when writing to your mum or dad, or whoever it might be. Try to write at least two pages. You might think that you don't have much to say, and maybe you won't. But equally you may find you have quite a few things you want to say. Don't feel bad about this; parents mostly do their best, but they don't always get it right and some get it very wrong indeed. Later, in your letter of thanks (see below), you can be grateful to them for all the good bits; but part of the process is recognizing the hurt.

I was in my thirties before I realized that I was really angry with my dad for dying when I was sixteen and leaving us five daughters and mum to cope on our own. Of course I couldn't be angry with him at the time for dying. Yet I *was* angry and my anger had no outlet. I only realized I was angry when I had a dream about him being alive and he told me he had not actually been dead all these years but living with another woman in Hong Kong. How strange the mind is. This strange dream enabled me to be angry with him, and – in the dream – I remember screaming at him about how angry he had made me for leaving us. After that I was able to accept how hard it had been not having a dad all those years, and I was finally able to let go of some of the hurt I had carried around with me.

In your letter you can express your anger and disappointment over something that perhaps the other person could not help, but it still left you with a negative emotion. The act of writing it down and acknowledging your feelings is incredibly therapeutic and will enable you to move forward on your journey.

A letter of thanks

This is a great way to give thanks for all the good things in your life and to focus on appreciation.

Many of us focus on what we don't have or feel that we are lacking in some way, when really we have many excellent qualities and many things to be grateful for in life. Writing them down in a letter is a way of refocusing our attention on the positive, to help celebrate the good in our lives rather than being self-critical or always seeing what we do not have. As Gandhi said:

'You must be the change you wish to see in the world.' That starts with you recognizing what is good in you and good in those people in your life.

There are several ways to do this, and I would urge you to find your own, but if you find it hard to start with yourself, begin by writing a letter to someone else who you might wish to thank. Try not to think about it too much – remember that no one is marking this and no one need ever see this letter. You can of course send it to the person you write about, but equally no one else need ever see it.

Forgiveness and compassion are an important part of this process. Write these letters from the most compassionate part of yourself, the part that is without petty judgment or criticism, the purest part. When I use the word 'pure', what I really mean is your higher self – the part of you that speaks the truth, not the part that has been indoctrinated by other people. Sometimes this voice can be hard to find, particularly if you have been in negative relationships or if you had parents who reinforced negative feelings. Accepting things about yourself and others is also very healing; there are some things about ourselves that we can change and there are others that we can't change. Accepting the parts we cannot change is an important part of any healing process.

Write as many letters as you want to as many people as you want; there is no limit on gratitude and compassion.

This form of letter writing is a really useful exercise and I urge you to try it. Whether you write in longhand or on the computer, let the words flow. At the end of the exercise reassess your feelings and emotions – you may find that you feel very different.

PART THREE
CHARTING
YOUR FERTILITY

For me, a woman's menstrual cycle is a window to her overall health. And of course it tells us so much about our fertility. My aim in this section is not only to show you how to interpret the key signals of your cycle, but also to show you what you can do to optimize your cycle. Charting your cycle, or writing a Fertility Diary, is a crucial part of understanding each phase. So I urge you to equip yourself with a notebook (or a smartphone app), to help you track the changes in your body each month.

The average menstrual cycle is around 28 days, with ovulation occurring around day 14. Don't worry if your cycle is shorter or longer than this; what we are aiming for is regularity to within a couple of days each month. Menstruation generally occurs 14 days after ovulation, but not always.

The menstrual cycle comprises four phases: during your period; the follicular phase pre-ovulation; ovulation; and the luteal phase before your period begins again. You will be potentially fertile for a few days during each cycle around ovulation. Eggs live for roughly 14 hours after being released, and sperm can stay alive and active in the body for two or three days. But at this point I would urge you to start thinking about your whole cycle, as each phase is related to all of the others and so focusing all your energy on just a couple of days around ovulation might mean you miss the key factor – be it big or small – that might optimize your fertility.

My aim as a practitioner is always to restore the body's rhythm and regularity and to ensure the smooth flow of Qi (energy), as well as to calm the mind. The idea is that if you remind the body what it is meant to be doing, it will do what it needs to with a small amount of fine-tuning – a bit like a mechanic making a car run better.

THE MENSTRUAL CYCLE
(BASED ON AN AVERAGE 28-DAY CYCLE)

Days 1–5

- Oestrogen and progesterone levels are both low at the beginning of the cycle, which causes the beginning of the period.
- The pituitary gland then begins to make follicle-stimulating and luteinizing hormones (FSH and LH), which will stimulate growth of new follicles in the ovary.

Day 7

- One follicle will start to grow much more quickly and produce oestrogen.

Days 7–13

- High levels of oestrogen stimulate growth of the uterine lining, and fertile mucus is produced by the cervix.
- Oestrogen also causes the pituitary gland to produce LH, which stimulates enzymes and prostaglandins in the dominant follicle.

Day 14

- The follicle ruptures and the egg is released.

Days 15–25

- The ruptured follicle forms a corpus luteum, which produces hormones that stimulate the endometrium to secrete nutrients. This is the implantation phase if conception has taken place. It is thought that many pregnancies fail at implantation stage (see page 201), despite the emphasis in Western medicine on ovulation.

Days 25–28

- If implantation has not taken place, the corpus luteum dies and the levels of oestrogen and progesterone once again drop, causing the start of your period.

N.B. If the time between ovulation and the period is less than 14 days, this is known as luteal phase deficiency (see page 184).

OESTROGEN

- makes us look, feel and behave as women
- shapes our bodies and our emotions
- in women with the highest levels of the hormone, gives us large eyes, bigger lips and more shapely figures

PROGESTERONE

- calms the mind, decreases anxiety and depression
- aids sleep
- builds bones
- is a natural diuretic
- promotes peace and tranquillity

CHAPTER EIGHT
YOUR FERTILITY DIARY

In this chapter I will show you how you can chart your own cycle to really get to know your fertility. The key signs will be your temperature, the appearance of fertile mucus, your period and timing, i.e. how regular or not your period and/or ovulation is.

I have then set out a mini-plan for the four phases of the cycle as a reminder of what should ideally be happening when, along with the diet and lifestyle advice that I generally recommend to everyone. Finally I have outlined the main things that I see going out of kilter with the cycle, including what you and the experts can do about each of these conditions.

CHARTING YOUR TEMPERATURE

Measuring your basal body temperature (BBT) is crucial if you really want to understand your cycle in terms of fertility and knowing the best days for potential conception.[56] The BBT is most accurate if taken at the same time each day before rising, using the same thermometer (a digital thermometer is probably the easiest) and method each time. You can then mark the readings on your fertility chart starting from the first day of your period (see page 152 for examples).

On day 1 of your cycle/period, the normal BBT is approximately 36.5°C (97.7°F) and should remain constant until just before ovulation, when you should observe a sudden drop. After ovulation, the temperature should quickly rise again and reach a peak within two to three days. There should be a difference in temperature between the pre-ovulation readings and post-ovulatory readings of at least 0.4°C. If the difference is less, we can look at whether this may indicate an incomplete pre-ovulation or post-menstruation phase. The temperature readings will then drop back down towards the first day of your next cycle.

It's important to take these readings over the entire cycle. Ideally I recommend that women spend four months observing and then fine-tuning to find their natural cycle. Often over a few days you will see your temperature readings go up and down, but this doesn't necessarily signify ovulation. And unstable emotions during the follicular phase can result in a seesaw of temperature readings. You need to look at the full cycle to recognize the big spike that occurs post-ovulation and the drop on day 1 of your next period.

Overleaf is an example of how the temperature chart might look. You can note alongside your BBT any other physical changes that occur.

Some women find that taking their temperature every day can feel a bit too controlling and obsessive. It can also be demoralizing if you aren't seeing the changes in temperature that signal ovulation. You might prefer to stick with checking your cervical fluid as described below. Alternatively, some companies provide a service whereby they are able to automatically check your temperature each day and then send you the results and possible interpretations of your BBT chart (see Resources for details). If you do choose this route, then I would try out the diet, mind and lifestyle advice I've included in the book for a couple of months alongside the charting, as you might see positive changes this way.

OBSERVING CERVICAL FLUID DURING YOUR CYCLE

Whether your cycle is long or short, regular or irregular, if you are experiencing that very slippery, egg-white-like mucus, your body is signalling that eggs are developing and being released. And along with the BBT, which will give a clear indication that you have ovulated, you can begin to develop a really good awareness of your fertility throughout the month.

After ovulating, the egg can be fertilized for up to 14 hours afterwards. And the mucus your body creates also helps to keep sperm alive before the egg is released (at other times of the month the natural acids in the vagina will kill sperm cells). So you can count any day when you feel this slippery mucus as a fertile day.

Temperature Chart

Name

Month: SEPTEMBER | OCTOBER

Date: 14 15 16 17 18 19 20 21 22 23 24 25 26 27 28 29 30 1 2 3 4 5 6 7 8 9 10 11 12 30 31 32 33 34 35 36 37 38

Day of cycle: 1 2 3 4 5 6 7 8 9 10 11 12 13 14 15 16 17 18 19 20 21 22 23 24 25 26 27 28 29

Temperature (°C):
38.2
38.1
38.0
37.9
37.8
37.7
37.6
37.5
37.4
37.3
37.2
37.1
37.0
36.9
36.8
36.7
36.6
36.5
36.4
36.3
36.2
36.1
36.0
35.9
35.8
35.7
35.6
35.5

OVULATION

THERMAL SHIFT

Commence new chart

Bleeding: X X X X X X

Intercourse: X X X X X X X X X X X

Your cervical mucus changes throughout the cycle in terms of how much you can feel, the colour and texture. For most women the typical observations are as follows:

- Right after your period, you may either have a rather dry vaginal sensation, or you may notice a slight moisture but little fluid, or that it is sticky in nature but not wet.
- For the next few days, you may notice the fluid is creamy and feels almost cool. It might be quite wet, and equally the vaginal sensation will be wet too.
- The most fertile fluid, which is present for the few days around ovulation (days 11–14 on average) is like raw egg white in texture – slippery and very stretchy, usually clear and very lubricating. This lubricating sensation is a crucial sign that you are at your most fertile, and it may continue for a few days. It is not the same as sexual lubrication, but something you can simply feel throughout the day. This fertile mucus is crucial, as it protects the sperm from the acid environment of the uterus.
- After ovulation, fluid will tend to be more dry in texture, slightly yellow, sticky and cloudy.
- Swimming can dry up the mucus for a few hours, but it doesn't stop you being fertile so it is fine to go ahead and swim. Check beforehand to see whether the mucus is present.
- If you have a short cycle, the mucus may appear towards the end of your period or very soon after.

WHAT TO NOTE

At the beginning of the day chart your basal body temperature, and at the end of each day write in your Fertility Diary your observations of how you are feeling physically, the consistency and appearance of cervical mucus, and how you are feeling mentally and emotionally. The following prompts are designed to help you, but of course feel free to write whatever you like.

Things to observe:
- physical observations, like cramps during your period, headaches, cervical fluid, etc.

- heightened feelings, or perhaps an absence of feelings
- memorable dreams and sleep patterns
- strong intuitive moments
- desire for intimacy, or perhaps the desire to be alone feeling sexual, or not feeling interested in sex
- how you feel about life and work
- how you are getting on with others
- whether you are in active mode or procrastinating over things
- whether you are worrying over little things or feeling at ease

From reading all the previous chapters, you will already have a good idea of where you might be able to make some tweaks in your lifestyle or diet to improve things. You might also be seeing clues that might point to fertility issues that may need addressing, whether directly related to hormone imbalances, or as a result of possible conditions like endometriosis or PCOS. I hope that as you observe your actual cycle (and I would encourage you to do this for a few months, if time is on your side), you will see how you can put the different parts of the fertility puzzle together – diet, mindfulness, exercise – in the best way for you as an individual. I'd encourage you to spend a bit of time writing down your plan of action, or highlighting a few days in your diary for when being observant of your cycle can make a big difference.

WORKING OUT YOUR FERTILE WINDOW

There is a simple calculation you can do that, in addition to the BBT readings and observation of cervical mucus, will help you identify your potentially fertile days during your cycle.

You need to work out your longest cycle over, say, the past six months and also your shortest cycle. Then subtract 20 from the shortest cycle and 10 from the longest. For example, if you had a cycle of 26 days as your shortest and 30 days as your longest, you would subtract 20 from 26 and 10 from 30 to give you 6 and 20. This is your fertility window: you would be potentially fertile from day 6 through to day 20. In reality, you will only be fertile for a few days in each month, but this calculation shows how much that can vary from month to month. It's a useful reminder not to always put all the focus around day 14.

INTERPRETING YOUR CYCLE

At the end of your cycle, as the next begins, take a step back to reflect on the patterns in your observations, both physical and emotional. This may take a few cycles to grasp, and that's OK; it's better to take your time than to jump too quickly to any strong conclusions. But once you do see the pattern, I hope you'll feel at ease with your cycle and know when you tend to feel energized and creative versus when you need to be still and take a little time out.

You will begin to understand how different foods affect you both positively and negatively during the four phases of your cycle, and likewise what types of exercise are helpful and at what times (and when to give the gym a miss for the night). Many of my patients tell me that after just a few months, 'problems' such as strong cramps, exhaustion and extreme mood swings fade away. They still experience the distinct phases of their cycle, like ovulation and pre-menstruation, but in a more balanced way that is no longer something to be dreaded.

WHEN TO HAVE SEX?

Understandably, many of my patients are fixated on this question. One of the hardest aspects of my job is talking to couples about sex, not because I feel uncomfortable, but because I think it's so hard to be prescriptive about it. What I really want to say is: don't try to time it – have sex whenever you feel like it. However, there are issues around this: the first is that some couples find it hard to fit sex into their lives, and also it is definitely important to understand your fertile window and try to have sex more often around this time.

If I had to be prescriptive, I would say that it's important to have sex throughout the month once every one or two days. If that is not possible, then I would suggest that you should increase to that frequency during days 14–16 in a 28-day cycle (earlier for shorter cycles), as the best time to have sex is most likely to be two days before ovulation. If your cycle isn't regular you will need to make this window bigger. But please don'r become overly fixated – regular sex throughout the month is the overall message here.

There is some perceived wisdom that men need to conserve their sperm over the month, but this is definitely not the case. If a man has sex regularly throughout the month, he will be producing newer, 'fitter' sperm all the time. Men produce three million sperm per day, so having regular sex (or indeed masturbating) means that during the fertile window you are more likely to produce sperm that can make it through the cervix to fertilize the egg. If as a couple you are having little sex, or waiting for a few days around ovulation, you may be reducing your chances of conception, as the sperm will be older and of lesser quality. And it might be worth bearing in mind that on average there is only a 2 per cent chance of conception each time a couple has sex.

MINDFULNESS THROUGH THE CYCLE

I want to encourage you to be mindful about your cycle: to begin to engage in it in a positive way and gently observe the physical and emotional changes you experience throughout the month. Give attention to this part of you that is at the heart of your fertility and try to become more familiar with it. Try to set aside some time each day just to relax and observe or record how you are feeling. You don't need to do anything; this is simply paying attention with no judgment. It sounds easy, but don't be surprised if it takes a little practice; it is often hard for us to do things that have no specific end gain.

At this stage I want you to practise observing and feeling.

Observing and feeling

Set aside five minutes of the day to be completely alone and look inward. I want you to pay attention to subtle details. Perhaps note how you are breathing and how your body feels – do you ache anywhere? How do you feel emotionally? Are you hot or cold? How do your abdomen and your breasts feel? Note all of these things and then let them go. Don't look for meaning in them; at this stage, it is simply about being aware and in the moment. We often get so caught up in following someone else's 'plan' that we forget to listen to what our own body is saying.

See this as a practice: in other words, the more you do it, the better you will get. It's amazing how distanced we can become from our body and mind when we decide we are ready for a baby, and instead start to become fixated on that very short time around ovulation. I want you to let go of any feelings of anxiety or obsession and just feel.

Perhaps through the process of being quiet, emotions may come up that you would like to address, or these feelings may dissolve naturally just by being allowed to come to the surface.

I think it is worth keeping in mind that some days are harder, while on other days things just seem to flow and be aligned without effort. I have learnt that we should not hide from pain, because it is from pain that transformation can happen. Menstrual pain tells us a great deal about what is going on for us, so it's important to pay attention rather than instantly pop a painkiller. Equally, many girls may celebrate the fact they have not had a period in months, but we need to listen to these messages and understand the clues they offer to our bodies and our fertility.

The emotional types throughout the cycle

Each emotional type will respond differently to the exercise of charting their fertility.

- All Heart types will be full of optimism and engage in this new task with renewed hope and enthusiasm, sure that it will deliver some answers that will ultimately bring about a baby. You are the opposite to the Visionary in a way, as you prefer fantasy to reality and sometimes you do much better through not knowing everything; it means that you can remain in your optimistic and extraordinary bubble, where nothing mundane ever happens. You may find focusing on the ordinary just a little too dull. as reality can tend to bring you down.
- The Thinker, who is better at organizing everyone else, will find the focus on them to be difficult and it may make them feel uncomfortable. A Thinker might say: 'It's so much better to be thinking about someone else; if I have to think about myself, I tend to end up worrying.' I encourage you to try it, though, as it is good for you to do things regularly and to form some healthy habits. You may particularly benefit from the act of regularly taking your temperature.
- The Perfectionist will love the precise discipline of plotting and planning the menstrual cycle and when to have sex. Just be careful not to make it all a bit too mechanical, because it's easy to lose the passion and fun when you are submersed in all of this.
- The Visionary will enjoy the idea of charting the cycle, because it may bring them closer to discovering the 'truth'; it will be like a window inside themselves. For the Visionary, knowledge is

power. I think this is a very useful exercise for you, as it will help you gain knowledge of your body that will either put your mind at rest or confirm that something does need addressing. You will be OK with that: whether the news is good or bad, you take it all the same way – it is the knowing that is important to you.

- The Planner will of course enjoy planning various 'things to do' throughout the cycle, although their impatience may get in the way of taking their temperature and monitoring the cycle. Give it a go, although it may not be for you – I suspect you might want to throw the diary out of the window if it frustrates you too much! Try to approach this in a meditative fashion and with a free and easy attitude. The regularity will do you good.

CHAPTER NINE
YOUR CYCLE PHASE BY PHASE

PHASE 1: DURING YOUR PERIOD

The bleed begins on day 1. If your period starts in the afternoon or evening, count the next day as day 1. The period should start 14 days after ovulation; if it occurs anything less than 12 days afterwards, it might be that you have a luteal phase deficiency (see page 184). Make a note if the bleed comes straight away or in dribs and drabs. Note the colour and consistency. Are there clots? Is there pain? Is it a sharp pain or a 'dragging down' feeling? Is there a change in your bowel movements? By day 2 or 3, the blood should be more of a bright red and flowing well without clots. Clots and pain are a sign to me of Stagnation of the Blood, i.e. it is not flowing freely enough. This is why I encourage foods that move the Blood during this first phase, and then foods that nourish the Blood through the rest of the cycle. Taking on the suggestions for mindfulness and exercise throughout the cycle will also help to balance things out.

Make a note of how many days you bleed for. The duration of the period is quite varied from woman to woman, but if it is less than three days and bleeding is light, this may indicate that the endometrium is not thickening properly, or that there may be Stagnation or retention and the lining is not shedding properly.

If the bleeding starts very quickly and is very red, this is a sign to me of Heat in the body (see page 247).

Also note if the flow stops and starts, or if the period stops altogether and then returns after one or two days. This would indicate to me that there may be a Stagnation in the flow of Blood and that the body is not shedding the endometrium smoothly. Warmth and gentle movement may help, as does acupuncture and increasing Blood-moving foods (page 65), which I encourage for all. Many women find warmth helpful during their period, particularly if they tend towards feeling the cold (a sign of which is dark and clotted blood). Don't use tampons at night, and if possible reduce tampon use during the day, because they can cause blood clots to travel back up into the uterus.

During your period I want you to pay attention to all these things above, and also to imagine that the lining of your uterus is shedding completely and fully. This is the cleansing phase: getting rid of the old before constructing the new. It is a time for quiet contemplation, for simplicity and peace. I always think it is valuable to make time for yourself during this phase and not to be too energetic or extrovert. Conserve your energies and honour your mood, because often the things that come up at this time are being brought to your attention by a wise part of yourself. I know that for some women the arrival of the period can bring a moment of grief too, as it can represent another month in which pregnancy has not occurred. Remember that with the period comes the promise of the chance to start again.

If your period doesn't arrive, or if it comes weeks later than your cycle tells you it should, do look at your emotional state. Your Heart controls your Blood and so your periods are intrinsically linked to your emotions.

If the BBT does not drop at the start of the menstrual flow and the tongue is purple with distended veins underneath, this can be the sign of quite severe Blood Stagnation, perhaps from a previous injury, miscarriage, retained products from a pregnancy or Asherman's (page 17). It would be worth having this checked out medically if your history warrants it.

UNDERSTANDING YOUR MENSTRUAL SYMPTOMS

I encourage all women, whatever their age, to observe their monthly period and learn from it. It is possible to identify a few key imbalances by observing your menstrual symptoms, and this will help you understand what you need to do in order to achieve balance. For example, if you feel that Stagnation of the Blood applies to you because you experience pain during your period and some of the blood is clotted, you can use some of the Blood-moving recipes or foods (see page 65). Perhaps your abdomen always feels cold: the remedy would be to include warming and more cooked foods. It seems too simple to be effective, but believe me: sometimes in this complicated world, a few simple messages to the body can have far-reaching effects.

I've set out below what some particular symptoms may mean.

Menstrual blood
- lack of blood: Blood Deficient
- heavy bleed: Heat (if very red) or weakness of Qi
- watery bleed: Blood or Yin Deficient
- clotted bleed: Blood Stagnation
- purple: Cold
- blackish: Blood Stagnation

Pain
- before the period: Qi Stagnation
- during the period: Blood Stagnation
- after the period: Blood Deficient
- pain relieved by warmth: Cold
- stabbing and severe: Blood Stagnation
- pain at ovulation: Damp (sometimes combined with Heat)

Regularity
- early: Heat or Deficiency of Qi
- late: Cold, Blood Stagnation or Blood Deficient
- irregular: Qi Stagnation

General signs of Qi Stagnation tend to include irritability before the period, with distended breasts and abdomen, often alternating between constipation and loose stools.

Water retention prior to the period tends to be because the Yang of the body is weak and the body needs warming from foods, herbs or acupuncture with hot needles.

PROBLEMS THAT MAY ARISE
No periods (amenorrhoea)
There are times in a woman's life, such as after childbirth, after a shock or a trauma or a change in environment, when her periods may temporarily stop. This is perfectly normal, and periods should resume after a month or two. However, if the time without a period is prolonged (three months or more), it is important to let your GP know.

Causes
- Amenorrhoea may be the side effect of certain medication; also, when you stop taking oral contraceptives it can take three to six months for regular periods to resume.
- Blood Deficiency: I see this a great deal, and it could be due to a heavy blood loss, either during labour, or through heavy periods or any other form of blood loss.
- An excess of overly sweet and sugary foods and alcohol: these tend to lead to Stagnation in the body and can really slow down or prevent the release of an egg.
- Fibroids or cysts.
- Emotional frustration or sadness: these feelings are common while trying to conceive and can actually end up contributing to the problem. Trying to time sex to the day and the hour can actually lead to you stopping yourself from ovulating. Feeling sad and frustrated may be temporary, or it may be more deep set.
- Stress can cause periods to stop, as can low body weight or excessive exercise.

- Lack of rest: for some women, missed periods are down to always being 'on the go', never getting adequate rest and running on empty for a long time. Many women overwork without taking adequate rest. This can apply to working long hours, but it can also apply to over-exercising.

Hormonal causes

- Polycystic ovary syndrome (PCOS; see page 194).
- Thyroid malfunction: overactive or underactive thyroid function may cause menstrual irregularities.
- Premature menopause: for some women, the ovarian supply of eggs is smaller and so menstruation stops before the age of forty.

Gynaecological causes

- Uterine scarring (Asherman's; see page 17): this can occur after Caesarean section, dilation and curettage, or treatment for fibroids.
- Vaginal structure: an obstruction of the vagina may block the flow of blood from the uterus and cervix.

Treatments

- You may need to have an operation to remove fibroids or cysts.

Toolbox

- In terms of your menstrual chart, it is important to focus your attention on the follicular phase (see page 166).
- Much can be done to help Blood Deficiency through diet. Include foods from the list on page 65, and also add beetroot and other Blood-nourishing foods to your diet.
- Rest is also important, so make sure you are getting plenty of good rest and that you are sleeping well (see page 178).
- Blood-moving foods (see list on page 65) may help with fibroids and cysts, and so will staying active and keeping the abdomen warm.
- Make time to address emotional problems or stress if the feelings are overwhelming. Ask yourself what the emotion is behind your lack of period. Issues of fear in relation to growing up or moving on are common.

- It is important to clean up the diet and avoid sugary foods and alcohol.

Painful periods (dysmenorrhoea)

For many women, the beginning of their period is a little inconvenient, while for others it makes them feel terrible for the first couple of days with painful cramping. This is why we look to build a smooth cycle throughout, because if we concentrate on improving the qualities of Blood, we will be less likely to suffer symptoms like menstrual cramps or mood swings later in the cycle.

Causes

- Endometriosis can be a cause of painful, heavy or irregular periods (see page 191).
- Oestrogen dominance may be a factor.
- Painful periods can be made worse by being upset around ovulation, a knock-on effect that also tends to be a part of PMS (see page 181).
- Cramps may also be the result of Cold in the body (see page 246), hence the relief provided by a hot-water bottle. Alternatively it may be a sign that the Blood isn't building well through the cycle or moving well during the period.
- In my clinic, pain of any kind means Stagnation. If the pain moves, it is Stagnation of the Qi or energy (see page 243); if the pain is fixed, it is the more serious type of Stagnation of the Blood (see page 244). Another way to tell if it is this Stagnation of the Blood is to look underneath the tongue and see if the veins are purple and engorged.

Treatments

- Rather than treating the cause, most women with painful periods will be given painkillers to alleviate the symptoms. If the pain is very bad, conditions such as endometriosis will be investigated and treated.
- The contraceptive pill is often prescribed as a way to artificially balance out the cycle and again alleviate symptoms.
- Acupuncture is excellent for painful periods.[57]

Toolbox
- Follow the advice for PMS (see page 182).
- Keep warm. Eat warming foods (see page 88) and avoid cold, raw foods.
- Some pain improves with heat: if this is the case for you, use a hot-water bottle.
- For others, the pain will improve with activity, so add a little exercise, like walking, to your day at regular intervals.
- Don't become too inactive, especially if the pain feels fixed and there are clots in the blood. If this is the case, focus on eating plenty of foods that are Blood-moving during your period (see page 65).
- If the pain feels much better for rest, you are Deficient rather than Stagnant in your Blood and Qi energy. Focus on the Blood-nourishing foods recommended on page 65, both after your period and throughout the cycle. And support your Qi with Qi-boosting foods (see page 81), and gentle tonifying exercise like yoga (see page 106).
- If you feel pain before your period starts, this is also an indicator of Stagnation of the Blood and Qi (see above).
- Massage your abdomen with a blend of aniseed, lavender and camomile essential oils. Do this once a day from three to five days before your period.
- Try an Epsom salts bath: add four cups of Epsom salts to the bath while it is running. Soak in the bath for about twenty minutes, and ideally rest afterwards too.
- Ask yourself what the emotion is behind your pain and nurture that part of you that needs attention.

Heavy periods (menorrhagia)

It is difficult to know what constitutes problematic heavy periods, but most women will know if their bleeding has gone significantly up or down.

Signs that your bleeding is unusually heavy would include:

- You are using an unusually high number of tampons or pads.
- You need to use tampons and pads together.
- You are experiencing blood flooding through to your clothes or bedding.

Causes
- endometriosis (see page 191)
- fibroids (see page 197)
- oestrogen dominance or hormone imbalance

Treatments
- If your periods continue to be heavier than normal for longer than one or two months, it is advisable to visit your doctor to rule out conditions such as fibroids (see page 197), which may be causing the excess bleeding.
- The most common medical treatment for menorrhagia is to prescribe one or more contraceptive pills to help balance your progesterone in the second half of the cycle, so that you don't produce such a thick lining of the uterus.

Toolbox
- If you try to balance your diet and lifestyle throughout your cycle, you may well find that you can do much to help balance things out yourself if it is hormones that are the cause.
- Eating plenty of Blood-nourishing and Blood-moving foods (see page 65), along with foods that support your Qi (see page 81), can be particularly helpful.
- If you experience excessive feelings of Heat during your cycle, then also look to include some cooling foods in your diet during the first half of the cycle. Eat plenty of salads, especially in the summer, plus leafy greens, beans and pulses, seaweed, seeds and nuts and fresh fish.
- Avoid caffeine and alcohol, as these are overstimulating.
- Avoid sour foods: they are astringent and tend to inhibit the flow of Blood.

PHASE 2: FOLLICULAR

After your period, it is important to nourish the Blood, as the growth part of your cycle begins again. In this phase the follicles are growing and producing increasing amounts of oestrogen. The endometrium is beginning to be constructed, hopefully to receive a fertilized egg (embryo) in the luteal phase. Imagine that you are growing healthy follicles from which you will produce an egg! It is vital to nourish yourself at this stage, as a good-quality egg will become an embryo strong enough to make it to implantation and become a healthy foetus.

If your BBT does not drop as ovulation approaches, this may indicate some retained blood, so continue with the Blood-moving foods. It is important that the lining of the uterus sheds properly, so that a healthy new one can be constructed.

As you near ovulation, you will begin to produce cervical mucus, the magical substance that will help the sperm on its difficult journey through the cervix and help it arrive in time to fertilize the egg. So this is the time to build up the essential secretions needed for creating a fertile and receptive environment around the time of ovulation. In this phase it is important to choose foods that support the gentle build-up towards ovulation, so opt for Yin-nourishing foods. (We also include Blood-nourishing foods after our period, so that we use the full length of the cycle to build the quality of our endometrial lining.) It is best to avoid overstimulating foods during this phase, and coffee is a really bad idea. Hydrating foods, especially soups and teas, are very helpful at this stage. Traditionally in China women drink soup made with Blood-nourishing herbs such as *shan yao* (yam), *sheng jiang* (ginger), *gou qi zi* (lycium berries) or *long yan rou* (logan fruit) during this post-menstrual phase.

If you notice you have little or no mucus (the stretchy, egg-white like fertile mucus should be present for three days), see page 169 for extra tips on improving fertile mucus. We are looking to create a slow and gentle build-up to the point of the egg being released. This is especially the case for quite a few slightly older women, or if you have a short cycle. We don't want the egg to release too early in the cycle before it is mature.

It's interesting that this is often a time of the month when women feel particularly productive or creative, as though we are in tune with what is going on physically. Our lifestyle should ideally reflect this feeling, but try not to suddenly rush around or spend endless hours in front of the computer. Build up your energy and activities gently. This is all about potential – the potential that one egg holds is quite amazing.

For the vast majority of women, the length of the cycle depends on the length of the follicular phase, i.e. how long it takes to grow the follicle and release a mature egg. If your cycle is 28 days, this would be around 14 days;

for women with a 35-day cycle it is likely to be around 21 days; and for a 24-day cycle it will be 10 days (although some women do have a short luteal phase between ovulation and their period; see page 184). It is more important for your periods to be regular than for them to last exactly 28 days. Irregular periods can indicate that other conditions may be a factor, like endometriosis (see page 191), PCOS (see page 194), fibroids (see page 197) or thyroid problems (see page 199).

PROBLEMS THAT MAY ARISE
Short follicular phase

If the follicular phase, i.e. from the first day of the period to ovulation, is consistently only 9 or 10 days, the egg may be being released too early, when it is not fully developed. The body loses energy as well as blood during this period and so needs enough time to replenish these. I will look for signs of either too much Heat in the body, or too little Yin, or a combination of both.

Signs of Heat include:

- heavy periods
- bright-red blood
- prone to fevers
- prone to acne
- lack of urine
- thirsty all the time
- dry stools
- feeling 'charged'
- can have a quick temper and find it difficult to relax
- tendency to binge when it comes to eating and drinking

Signs of not enough Yin include:

- feeling hot and dry in the body
- not much fertile mucus
- scanty periods
- feeling restless or anxious
- often wiry, with prematurely ageing skin
- overworked and stressed

Toolbox
- It is a good idea to start building the Blood (see page 65 for Blood-nourishing foods) and Yin (see below) a little earlier than usual and focus on this second phase for a while, to see if it is possible to lengthen the time between the period and ovulation.
- Beneficial herbs include floradix and chlorella.
- Whether you observe feelings of Heat and/or Yin Deficiency, avoiding alcohol and caffeine will help for both. Recreational drugs also play havoc with Heat.
- Cut down on greasy and sugary foods.
- Have acupuncture to regulate the cycle.
- Develop ways to relax and calm your mind; yoga and meditation will be especially beneficial.

HEAT AND FERTILITY PRESERVATION

Warmth is important to activate the body and to support physiological function. Problems arise when there is sustained Heat over too long a period of time or when the Heat is excessive. In excess, Heat dries up fluids, can cause inflammation, redness and agitation. Think about how you would like your ovaries and your follicles to be and how you would like your endometrium to be: warm, yes, but definitely not dry and agitated.

Heat to the testicles is known to damage sperm; this is why the testicles hang outside the body, to keep their precious cargo of sperm healthy and cool. The ovaries, however, are buried deep within the body, protecting their precious treasure. But just like sperm, it appears that eggs do not like extreme heat either. Below are a list of things you may not have thought about that also generate Heat within the body and can potentially cause problems.

- excessive consumption of spicy foods
- excessive consumption of fried and greasy foods

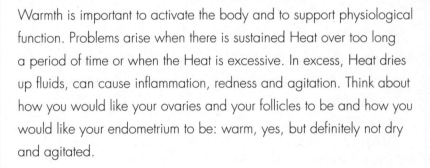

- excess alcohol (spirits and red wine are heating in smaller amounts)
- coffee and caffeine
- keeping emotions pent up
- emotional stress and anxiety
- environmental factors and endocrine disruptors
- unresolved illness, low-grade infections and pathogens retained in the body over a long period of time
- drugs and cigarettes
- radiation
- excessive exercise

Studies have shown that in warm climates, egg quality is reduced after a particularly warm spell.[58] The findings suggest that the heat affects the early development of the follicles and that the effects can last for some months. If this is the case in hot weather, it is likely that all extreme heat sources could potentially affect egg quality in the same way. Research looking at the effects of heat during ovarian stimulation have also concluded that it can reduce the number of eggs collected and impair quality.

It is likely that these findings mirror the Chinese medicine theory that the Yin of the body is vital to maintaining good fertility. When we live excessively, work long hours, don't take adequate rest and are exposed to high levels of toxins both in our food and drink and in our environment, we damage our body's natural protective defenses. Perhaps heat and toxins have a damaging effect on the follicular fluid (the most Yin of all fluids) and prevent it from being able to fulfill its role of protecting and nourishing the egg.

Toolbox

- Identify where the Heat sources are coming from: are they emotional, a stressful job, baby-making anxiety or dietary? These

are areas you can do something about. If the source is emotional,
see Fertility Mindfulness (page 116) and if dietary, see In the
Fertility Kitchen (page 54).

- Get checked out for low-grade infections; see a GP but also an
  acupuncturist or herbalist who can readdress any deep-seated
  energetic imbalances causing Heat.
- Environmental heat and endocrine disruptors are more tricky; some
  factors we can do something about and some we can't control.
  Try to keep your environment as free of toxins as possible and use
  natural products (toiletries, cleaning products, organic foods where
  possible). Keep computers and electrical equipment out of your
  bedroom. I was told once to keep a jar full of Epsom salts under
  my bed. I am not sure if this works, but I do it anyway!

Long follicular phase

A long follicular phase isn't thought to be too much of a problem for most
women, but we always try to tweak things in the diet and lifestyle departments
if possible, to encourage a 14-day follicular phase.

Causes

A delay in ovulation may be because the egg isn't getting enough nutrients to
mature on time, or for some women may be related to being very stressed, as
heightened anxiety or frustration can prevent or delay ovulation.

Slow follicular development may be due to low oestrogen levels, unstable
FSH levels and/or low levels of the anti-Müllerian hormone (AMH); these
are signs of low ovarian reserve and a lack of Yin.

Sometimes the BBT will rise as if ovulation has occurred, but this does
not guarantee that an egg has been released. Checking the cervical mucus can
help determine this. If there is concern, an FSH test will be able to determine
if ovulation is taking place (see page 32).

When I see patients, I look to see if there is a great deal of Dampness in
the body (see page 245) which is slowing the release of the egg, or if there is
a high level of Stagnation in the pelvic cavity, including digestion.

Toolbox

- It is nearly always important to nourish the Blood in the follicular phase (see page 65 for foods).
- As you get closer to ovulation, increase your activity. This will prevent Stagnation in the abdominal cavity.

PHASE 3: OVULATION

In a 28-day cycle, ovulation will normally occur on day 14, but this can vary from woman to woman. Remember, a calm mind will help you release an egg. Some distension or mild pain in the abdomen is common, but stronger pain is something we can address (see page 176). Libido is usually raised at this time of the month, and often if we listen to and feel our responses rather than trying to orchestrate everything, then our body will tell us when is the optimum time to have sex (see page 155). An increase in lovemaking needs to start several days prior to ovulation to increase the chances of the sperm meeting the egg.

You should be able to observe the presence of the fertile cervical mucus during these days around ovulation (like raw egg white). After ovulation the fluid will tend to be more dry and sticky in texture. And you should observe a sudden drop in your BBT just before ovulation. It should then quickly rise to a peak a couple of days later.

It is so important to be relaxed and 'in the moment' during this phase. As we have seen, the mind is very important when it comes to your overall cycle and in particular around the ovulation stage. Some women can actually struggle to release an egg if they are very emotionally tense. If you find that you feel tense, try a gentle breathing exercise (see page 183).

Many conditions I see in my clinic such as amenorrhoea, dysmenorrhoea or irregular bleeding improve once ovulation is promoted and optimized, which I do by strongly activating Qi energy.

Around the time of ovulation, it is very helpful to support the digestion and keep your energy nicely topped up. A healthy balance of rest and also exercise is ideal. Think of what kinds of exercise make you feel energized rather than drained; for some women this might be a walk, while for others a workout in the gym is what you fancy. You want the energy in your reproductive area to be activated.

Flavoursome and fresh foods are just what you need (see page 81 for foods and recipes for this phase). If you are feeling very Damp or bloated, stick with foods that help to alleviate water retention (see page 82) and avoid the foods that make it worse like dairy and sugar. Foods that are good for the digestion will help to prevent any bloating, so plenty of aromatic herbs like basil, coriander and chives are good.

Focus on food as something that connects you and your partner and brings you together at this time. Bring all your senses to cooking and eating: be unhurried; enjoy your food; savour every flavour. It is advisable to eat light meals, and sticking mainly to vegetarian dishes is a good idea because they are easier on the digestion. Eat fewer starchy carbohydrates, especially in the evenings.

Keeping the body warm through movement and moxa (an external warming treatment offered by acupuncturists) are also good for helping to release an egg. However, if there is any bleeding during ovulation, this is a sign of Heat in the body and so avoid moxa, extra heat, coffee, alcohol and foods that are hot like chilli and strong spices. Make sure that you don't Stagnate; build movement into your day by walking some of the way to work, for example. Keep the Qi active.

PROBLEMS THAT MAY ARISE
Not ovulating
If you aren't having periods (see page 162), you won't be ovulating; irregular periods will also have an effect on ovulation. But some women have regular periods and still don't ovulate, which you can see by the lack of temperature change in the BBT (see page 150). And sometimes the BBT chart can show a rise in temperature, but an egg may not be released.

If you are using an ovulation testing kit, you may need to test in the morning and the evening to detect ovulation.

Causes
- If you're underweight, you may not be producing enough oestrogen to ovulate, as oestrogen needs body fat to be produced.
- Conversely, being overweight can cause you to have too much oestrogen in the body, which also can be very disrupting to your cycle.
- Polycystic ovary syndrome (PCOS; see page 194).
- Stress can affect ovulation. In Chinese medicine, anything that

affects the Heart and mind affects ovulation, which is why it is so important to feel calm around this time of the cycle.

• Age-related reduction in ovarian reserve (see page 31).

Treatments

Women taking clomifene (Clomid) to stimulate the release of an egg may find that it has the side effect of drying up the cervical mucus, which is needed to transport the sperm through the cervix to the egg (see below for natural ways to increase cervical mucus). If your period becomes lighter after taking Clomid, stop and take a month off. The best thing is to make sure you are scanned when taking Clomid (a transvaginal scan where a probe is inserted into the vagina to give a good view of the follicles growing on the ovaries and the thickness of the endometrium), or see a Chinese medicine practitioner to check that you are not Blood or Yin Deficient (Clomid is less likely to help if either of these are the case and they are best addressed first).

Toolbox

Assessing the quantity and quality of cervical mucus gives important clues about a woman's fertility. You may notice a lack of fertile cervical mucus at the time around which you should be ovulating. This may be due to a number of factors:

• Coming off the pill recently: it can take a couple of cycles for your body to re-adjust.
• Vaginal lubricants can alter the pH of your mucus membranes and make your vaginal environment hostile to sperm. There are now lubricants available that are the same pH as the vagina.
• Anti-inflammatory medications, antihistamines, and antibiotics may also affect the quality of fertile mucus.
• Too many heating foods (see page 88) and not enough Yin (see page 10) in the body.
• If you are ovulating but not producing the right kind of fertile mucus, you may be referred for the assisted conception treatment IUI (intrauterine insemination). In this process the sperm is inserted straight into your uterus and so bypasses the need for the mucus.

TIPS FOR PRODUCING MORE CERVICAL MUCUS

- Drink lots of water (not from the fridge).
- Include Yin-nourishing foods in your diet in the first half of the cycle (see page 72).
- Avoid antihistamines and cough or cold medicines, as these often have the effect of drying up mucus membranes. However, some cough medicines contain expectorants that thin mucus, and it is thought that these medications might actually increase cervical mucus. I personally think it is better to build up your Yin through diet and herbs.
- Avoid overly acidic foods, including too much red meat, refined sugar and saturated fats.

Supplements that may be of help include:

- L-Arginine may help to increase the fluidity and production of your mucus during ovulation.
- Lactobacillus acidophilus helps to keep healthy not only the gut environment but also the vagina.
- Calcium will make the pH of the cervical mucus less acidic and more sperm friendly.
- Evening primrose oil is an essential fatty acid that you can take after your period until ovulation to improve fertile mucus. But it is not recommended to take this supplement after ovulation, as it can cause mild contractions in the uterus and prevent implantation.

Pain on ovulation

About a fifth of women experience a degree of pain during ovulation, in the general area of the abdomen or on one side or the other. It is not normal, but is common. Usually it is just a mild annoyance, but for some the pain can be very uncomfortable. It is caused by the mature egg stretching the ovary membrane just before it is released and can last anything from between a couple of hours to three days. It can therefore be a useful indicator of when to increase the frequency with which you are having sex.

If the pain is severe, you may need to visit the hospital to rule out appendicitis. If you have bleeding alongside the pain, do visit your GP to investigate what might be causing the pain and bleeding.

Anti-inflammatory painkillers may be advised to alleviate the pain, although these can also have an adverse effect on the fertile mucus. Pain at ovulation is also well treated by acupuncture as it indicates Qi Stagnation.

Toolbox

- Apply a heating pad to the pelvic area to help alleviate the pain.
- Abdominal massage (by yourself or another) can be very helpful.
- Movement is important: belly dancing was born out of a wisdom that women need to move their midriff to avoid Stagnation. You might prefer to do 10 or 15 minutes of rebound exercise (such as trampolining), which is excellent at moving the Qi in the abdomen.

Spotting

Ovulation spotting: mild bleeding around mid-cycle at the time of ovulation.

Implantation spotting: when a fertilized egg implants there can be a small amount of blood 10–12 days after fertilization.

Causes

- cysts, polyps, infections of uterus or cervix
- chronic conditions such as diabetes or thyroid problems
- gonorrhea can cause spotting before the period, accompanied by pelvic pain
- more serious illnesses include cancer of the cervix or uterus (which is why regular cervical smear tests are so important)

In Chinese medicine, spotting can occur either because there is too much Heat (see page 247) or because the body's Qi is weak and not strong enough to hold the Blood. If there is some bleeding at ovulation, it is often because the Yin is too weak or the Liver energy is too strong.

Toolbox

- Both ovulation spotting and implantation spotting may be remedied by using agrimony tea (see Resources) or raspberry leaf tea.

- See page 81 for how to support Qi.
- Avoid stimulants (like caffeine and alcohol), rest and keep a calm, cool mind.

N.B. If you are at all concerned, do see your GP to rule out any medical conditions.

WHY MIGHT OVULATION STICKS REDUCE MY CHANCES OF CONCEIVING?

For a long time now I have been asking my patients to 'ditch the sticks' – to stop using ovulation testing kits (in all but a few cases). There are a number of reasons for this. First, I have noticed that most people who use them are using them to help them feel in control. The sticks make people believe that they can have sex just when the stick says so, and, hey presto, they will hit the jackpot. I also find they can cause stress in a relationship and reduce the amount of sex the couple has, sometimes to as little as twice a month.

The problem is that by reducing the frequency of sex, you are reducing the number of fresh sperm made every month – you need top-quality sperm to reach the goal. Second, you are reducing your chances of conceiving. It's really very simple: if you want a baby, you do need to prioritize sex and have regular sex throughout the month, rather than confining it to just a few days. So, again, I do tend to advise that you ditch the sticks.

However, for some patients who have very long or irregular cycles, ovulation sticks can be useful to identify the fertile time and whether you are ovulating.

PHASE 4: LUTEAL

This is the incubation phase, when you want to encourage implantation if fertilization of the egg has occurred. Successful implantation is likely to be a combination of a healthy, viable egg and a healthy, receptive endometrium. For all women, it's a time to keep warm. In terms of visualization, imagine the warmth of your body providing the perfect, receptive dwelling place for your baby.

This is the Yang phase; Yang can be likened to progesterone, in that it enables the embryo to be held securely in the uterus. When the Yin and the Blood are Deficient, the endometrium will be undernourished and may not be able to successfully implant an embryo. Many of these 'mini miscarriages' occur due to an inadequate luteal phase. If you are charting your BBT, see if your temperature rises and for how long.

Think about how you cook as well as what you eat: don't go for raw foods during this phase, but stick to more comforting soups, stews and mild spices. Warming foods are ideal (see page 88), as are Blood-nourishing foods (see page 65). You can enjoy a few more calories during this time of the month, so don't worry if your appetite increases – it's a healthy sign. Avoid very cold drinks and ice creams. And don't let yourself get too chilly. I am like a broken record with all my patients when I say never to go out with wet hair!

When I see patients in this phase, I am aiming to add warmth and keep the Yang high to 'hold' the pregnancy. In traditional Chinese texts there is a great deal of importance placed on a warm Womb. I often give my patients moxa during this phase, which is a wonderful warming technique for the abdomen. Getting enough good sleep is important too (see box).

TIPS FOR GETTING A GOOD NIGHT'S SLEEP

- Tryptophan-containing foods, like turkey, wholegrains, lentils, chickpeas, nuts and seeds are good, as this amino acid produces melatonin, which encourages sleep.
- Getting some exercise and daylight during the day helps your body to feel nicely tired and in need of a rest when night comes.

- Practising breathing exercises (see page 183) or meditation before bed can put you in a relaxed state.
- Keep anything electronic out of the bedroom.
- Don't work on the computer late in the evening, as this is over-stimulating.
- If you do like a coffee, have one mid-morning, but avoid it after midday as the effects can last right through into the evening and keep you awake. Herbal teas are good throughout the day, and camomile is particularly restful for the evening.
- Allow yourself to gently wind down throughout the evening; have a bath and relax. And try not to eat too late, so that your digestion doesn't have to work too hard while you are sleeping.

'Rest in natural great peace, this exhausted mind, beaten helpless by karma, and neurotic thoughts, like the senseless fury of the pounding waves, in the infinite ocean of samsara. Rest in natural great peace.'

Nyoshul Khen Rinpoche

Implantation

Implantation occurs about 8 to 10 days after ovulation. I think we underestimate just how many pregnancies fail at implantation. In my practice we always focus on making sure the endometrium is as healthy as possible (through good Blood flow) and on encouraging a receptive environment to help support implantation. Keeping the abdomen warm and being active goes some way to encouraging good movement and Blood flow to the endometrium. If the abdomen feels cold to the touch, you might want to warm the Womb by having a moxa treatment.

I find assessing the menstrual bleed and taking a detailed medical history is a good way of establishing if implantation might be an issue. Endometriosis (see page 191), fibroids (see page 197), polyps or scarring (see page 17) and blood-clotting disorders (see page 219) can all potentially hinder successful implantation and so they are best addressed individually. For example,

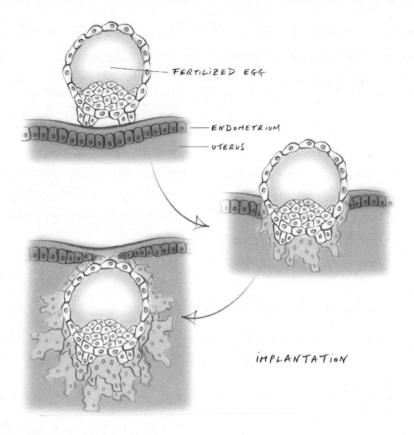

depending on the severity, for poor endometrial thickness we might look to nourish the Blood (see page 65), and for scarring and blood-clotting disorders we move the Blood (see page 65).

When there is bloating, irregular periods and/or digestive disturbance, it's a good idea to move the Qi around the body (see pages 81 and 106). And as with ovulation, a calm mind is also important to aid implantation. Try to relax as much as possible; if you feel tense, try a gentle breathing exercise (see page 183).

Allergies and yeast infections

When you are exposed to allergies, particularly over a long period of time, it can trigger an immune reaction which may hinder implantation. Most women will have a vaginal yeast infection, commonly thrush, at some point. This is where the fungus Candida albicans, which is often found in small amounts in the vagina, mouth, digestive tract and on the skin, increases in number and causes a yeast infection.

Yeast infections can create a hostile environment in the vagina for sperm, but they are usually easily treatable with medication. However, if the problem persists, this may lead to allergies that can trigger an autoimmune reaction. This has been linked to an increased risk of implantation failure (see page 220).

It is important to maintain high levels of good bacteria in the digestive tract to help keep candida at bay and help get back into a healthy balance after an infection. Good bacteria can be killed off by poor nutrition, the Pill, antibiotics, stress, pregnancy and diabetes. You can top up your levels with supplements.

One of the best ways to get rid of thrush is through a restrictive diet that cuts out all sugars, yeast, cow's milk, fruit (fresh or dried), nuts, all fermented foods, mushrooms, smoked or cured fish and meat, tea and coffee, carbonated drinks, malted foods, hot spices, artificial sweeteners, preservatives, salt and ground pepper. Phew: it doesn't seem like there will be much left to eat! But actually you can eat plenty of wholegrains like oats, quinoa, rice, herbs, mild spices, fresh fish, herbal teas, natural yoghurt, cottage cheese, butter, fresh vegetables, avocado, tomatoes, lemon, beans and pulses, organic lean meat, cold-pressed oils like olive oil, sunflower oil and flax seed oil, soya or rice milk. It is tough, so nutritionists often suggest that you are tested for Candida albicans before launching in to such a restrictive diet (see Resources for specialist help with nutrition).

PROBLEMS THAT MAY ARISE
PMS: Premenstrual syndrome

Our menstrual cycle does depend on a natural ebb and flow of hormones, and so changes in our mood and our body are to some degree normal and to be expected. However, many women nowadays experience a more extreme roller coaster of symptoms. I know from my clinical experience there is quite a bit that can be done to help make things much easier.

PMS can manifest in a variety of ways in the lead-up to your period:

- irritability and mood swings
- headaches
- dizziness
- sore breasts
- backache
- food cravings
- bloating

- lack of focus
- clumsiness
- difficulty sleeping
- depression

Causes

Western medicine hasn't yet pinpointed the exact causes of PMS, but the connection between fluctuations in hormones interacting with our brain's mood-controlling chemicals (serotonins) is thought to be a significant factor. This might also explain why stress, particularly around ovulation, can make PMS symptoms worse: the mind affects the body and the body affects the mind in a natural, sometimes virtuous, but sometimes vicious circle.

There is also a theory that a lack of essential fatty acids may be a factor. For tips on increasing these in your diet, see page 44.

If you are obese and don't exercise, or if you are a smoker, you are more likely to suffer from PMS. Try to lose weight and quit the cigarettes; this is a good idea for many reasons, not least to help overcome PMS.

Treatments

- Over-the-counter medications such as paracetamol, ibuprofen and aspirin may be advised for the relief of physical symptoms.
- Diuretics are also available if you suffer from bloating (see below for natural relief).
- Antidepressant medicines (SSRIs) can be helpful in helping the symptoms of PMS, but it won't be a surprise that most doctors aren't too keen to prescribe these medications apart from in cases of severe depression.
- Acupuncture can be very effective.

Toolbox

If you experience extreme symptoms of PMS, try the following advice from mid-cycle until the beginning of your period:

- Following a healthy diet of natural foods will help a great deal (see pages 62–4).
- Lose weight if you need to.
- Avoid spicy or fatty foods.

- Avoid refined sugar and refined grains such as white bread and pasta.
- Dandelion and fennel teas are natural diuretics for reducing bloating.
- Evening primrose oil supplements can be very helpful for some women.
- Bathe with essential oils such as lavender, camomile, geranium and orange.
- Take gentle and regular exercise.
- Try meditation or other relaxation techniques such as the 'humming-bee breath' (see box below, with kind permisssion from Uma Dinsmore-Tuli).

BHRAMARI: THE CALMING HUMMING-BEE BREATH

Sound and vibration can have a very calming effect on the body. I like to imagine the humming bee attracting a little soul to the Womb through its humming and vibration. Since anxiety is the enemy of fertility, I think this is a very useful exercise. This is to be done sitting up, cross-legged or in whichever sitting posture you find comfortable.

- First establish some gentle, regular, deep breathing.
- Then close the eyes.
- Raise the arms and draw the elbows out wide at shoulder height on the inhalation.
- Block the ears (with the heels of your hands, index fingers or thumbs, whichever works best for you).
- On the exhaling breath, make a humming sound. (The sound is felt more than heard, so don't strain to make it loud.) Focus your awareness of the sound vibrations in the centre of your chest.
- Allow for the sound to fade at the end of the exhalation, then start again.

This practice promotes feelings of tranquillity and is thought to connect the breath with the Womb. It is a very useful tool when you are feeling volatile or unsettled.

Luteal phase deficiency

Ideally the phase from ovulation to the next period should be 14 days, or a minimum of 12 days. If the luteal phase is too short, not enough progesterone is being produced and the lining of the uterus will therefore not provide the best environment possible for incubating a fertilized egg. So it is important to try to modify the length of this phase.

Causes

- Dietary deficiencies in B vitamins and magnesium may cause low levels of progesterone in some women.
- Chronic stress can affect the hormone balance throughout the cycle.
- Candida (see page 180) can make the situation worse.

Treatments

- Clomid works well for luteal phase deficiency, as it raises the temperature and lengthens the luteal phase.
- Progesterone suppositories can be beneficial.

Toolbox

- Again, this is a condition where cutting down on sugar and yeast in the diet is a very good idea, as any excess of candida can disrupt a healthy hormone balance.
- Getting enough B vitamins may be helpful for healthy progesterone levels. Foods high in vitamin B6 include blackstrap molasses (see my recipe for sticky ginger cake on page 93) and soya beans. Include flax seeds in your diet, as well as sweet potato. You can also make sure your daily vitamin supplement includes B6.
- Magnesium is also linked with low progesterone, so again make sure this is included in your daily vitamin supplement, along with foods rich in this mineral, particularly the leafy greens like spinach and kale, and almonds.
- You can also buy magnesium flakes for the bath, which feel lovely.

CYCLE AT A GLANCE

Phase 1: During your period

- Take things easy: go for a gentle walk rather than a high-energy workout.
- Try to get an early night.
- Look to include foods that encourage movement of Blood out of the body, i.e. complete discharge of the old endometrial lining (see page 65).

Phase 2: Follicular

- Stretchy, egg-white-like cervical mucus should appear a couple of days before ovulation.
- You should notice a drop in basal body temperature (BBT) just before ovulation.
- High-energy exercise is more suited to this phase.
- Be creative.
- Choose foods that support the gentle build-up towards ovulation, so Yin-nourishing and Blood-nourishing foods. It is good not to eat overstimulating foods during this phase, and coffee is a really bad idea. Opt for lots of soups and teas.

Phase 3: Ovulation

- The fertile mucus should continue to appear.
- After ovulation BBT will rise.
- Aim for a healthy balance of work, rest and play.
- Opt for the exercise you fancy, whether that's a nice walk or a session in the gym.
- Relaxation through meditation is excellent this time of the month.
- Support your Qi with oats in the morning and eat lightly in the evening.

Phase 4: Luteal

- BBT will continue to rise, peaking 2 or 3 days after ovulation, then decreasing towards the next period.
- Getting plenty of sleep is important.

- Never go out with wet hair.
- Avoid getting chilly and don't include too many cold foods and drinks in your diet.
- Keep warm when exercising.
- Enjoy a few more calories.
- This is the incubation phase and so we include plenty of warming, Yang-supporting foods.

PART FOUR
MANAGING YOUR FERTILITY

Quite often at my clinic I will see women in their thirties being diagnosed for the first time with conditions that they might have had for years. The problem with this is if you've had irregular cycles for fifteen years or more, it is harder to remedy. Although it's never too late to manage and treat these conditions, it can take time, so addressing gynaecological issues early in life can be extremely helpful when it comes to preserving your fertility. Women will suffer in silence, sometimes for years, taking painkillers to enable them to carry on as normal; or they may go long stretches of time without having a period at all, which might seem great when you're twenty but can pose a real problem when you want a baby.

COMMON CAUSES OF FEMALE INFERTILITY

- endometriosis (see page 191)
- polycystic ovary syndrome (PCOS; see page 194)
- fibroids (see page 197)
- thyroid problems (see page 199)
- premature ovarian ageing (see page 31)
- luteal phase deficiency (see page 184)
- ovulatory dysfunction (see page 178)
- damage to Fallopian tubes (see page 21)
- autoimmune diseases (see page 220)
- STDs (see page 21)

- genetics (see Ask Your Mum on page 18)
- age (see page 31)

At the back of the book I have included excellent books and websites for many of these conditions.

CHAPTER TEN
FERTILITY-RELATED CONDITIONS

ENDOMETRIOSIS

The endometrium lines the uterus and becomes thicker towards the end of the menstrual cycle to provide the right environment for the fertilized egg. If fertilization doesn't occur each month, the top layer breaks down and so we have our period. Endometriosis occurs when cells that should live inside the uterus migrate to other areas of the body, most commonly in the lower part of the pelvis, including the ovaries and Fallopian tubes. They might also migrate to the bladder or rectum, or even to the small intestine, kidneys or stomach. If left to develop, these patches or lesions can lead to intense pelvic pain and affect fertility. Women with severe endometriosis have lower pregnancy rates from IVF than women with tubal problems.

Main symptoms:
- pelvic pain and cramping
- pain during intercourse
- painful periods
- spotting between periods
- heavy bleeding
- irregular periods
- loss of large blood clots during menstruation
- bleeding from the bowel (this symptom should always be checked with your GP to rule out any other possible conditions)

- bowel discomfort
- bladder discomfort
- fertility problems
- depression or low moods
- feeling tired all the time
- migraines

Causes

The exact causes of endometriosis are as yet unknown, although there are a number of theories, including the following:

- Genetics: women who have a mother or sister with endometriosis are up to nine times more likely to develop the condition themselves. This is another very good reason to ask your mum about her own gynaecological history.

- Oestrogen imbalance: whether this is an actual cause or a factor in its progression, many women with endometriosis have a dominance of oestrogen, which causes a hormonal imbalance. This might be from the surge of oestrogen in the body during puberty or from xenoestrogens in the environment, for example in packaging and certain foods (see page 28).

- Menstruation cycle: women are at twice the normal risk of developing endometriosis if their cycle is less that 27 days on average and they also bleed for more than 7 days. Retrograde menstruation occurs when endometrial tissue flows up the Fallopian tubes and into the abdomen or bowel. Although it can happen to all women, in women with endometriosis the problem appears to be significantly worse and so may be a causal factor. The use of tampons can be a factor, as obstruction of the flow and exit of Blood from the cervix during the period is thought to be the main cause of retrograde menstruation. This is one of the reasons I always encourage my patients not to use tampons whenever possible, and also why I concentrate on improving the movement of Blood during the first phase of the cycle (see page 14).

- Delayed childbearing: there are suggestions that pregnancy does go some way to helping to protect the womb from conditions like endometriosis by giving our body a break from menstruation.

- Weakened immune system: like oestrogen dominance, a weak immune system might be both a cause of endometriosis and/ or a factor that makes it worse. The immune system will react to the condition as a threat, creating inflammation around the areas affected to try and protect the rest of the body. The immune system can end up becoming weakened as a result, which means a woman with the condition might then be less able to clear all of her menstruation blood effectively, so exacerbating the endometriosis – it can develop into a vicious circle.[59]

According to Henrietta Norton, a nutritionist who specializes in women's health conditions and author of *Take Control of Your Endometriosis* (see Resources), for most women the condition will tend to arise from a combination of some of all of these factors.

Medical treatments
- Progesterone or oral contraceptives may be prescribed to regulate and help promote and maintain a healthy menstrual cycle.
- Gonadotropin-releasing hormone analogues such as Zoladex: these are given as a monthly injection and cause a temporary reduction in oestrogen levels, which in turn causes temporary shrinkage of the endometriosis lesions.
- Surgery to remove areas of endometriosis has been shown to be successful and can improve natural fertility. A laparoscopy (also known as keyhole surgery) with laser ablation is often the preferred surgery, although the extent of endometriosis can sometimes demand more invasive surgery.

Toolbox
According to Henrietta Norton, there is much you can do to relieve the symptoms of endometriosis through diet and lifestyle. The aim is to improve immune function, digestive function, liver function (if the liver is too overworked, it can fail to remove all components of oestrogen from the bloodstream when it should) and hormone balance.

My main aim is to address Stagnation in the Blood. I think, if time allows, it is good to spend several months not trying to conceive while you follow a Blood Stagnation plan from ovulation until the end of your period, which

...ns not drinking alcohol, introducing Blood-moving foods (see page 65), using acupuncture and herbs, all of which are designed to move the Blood.[60] And you must nourish the Blood from after your period right through until ovulation (see page 65).

If endometriosis is extensive, you may well benefit from surgery; but then you should follow the programme outlined above for one or two months afterwards before trying to conceive.

Tips for all:
- Give up smoking.
- Avoid processed foods and sugar.
- Use a water filter to remove xenoestrogens (a reverse osmosis filter system is ideal, as it retains the trace minerals).
- Avoid plastic wrapping and plastic bottles, including cling film.
- Stress (see page 26) and lack of exercise can make the symptoms worse, so find ways to manage your stress levels and regularly take a form of gentle exercise that you enjoy.
- Get plenty of vitamin D, which is good for your immune system, by going outside in the natural daylight.
- Try not to use tampons.
- To relieve pain, apply a heating pad.
- Have a bath with Epsom salts. This helps relieve pain and also restores pH balance in the body, which reduces inflammation.
- Dandelion and nettle teas are good for the liver.
- Avoid excessive alcohol to help restore good liver function.
- Colonic irrigation can help cleanse the bowel.
- Dry skin brushing (see page 127).
- Sleep well (see page 178).
- Try meditation.

POLYCYSTIC OVARY SYNDROME (PCOS)

It is thought up to one in ten women of reproductive age are affected by polycystic ovary syndrome, or PCOS, a condition related to hormone imbalance. The main problems associated with PCOS are menstrual cycle disturbances, including irregular or absent periods, weight gain that is difficult to shift, excess hair growth and skin conditions like acne.

Usually during your menstrual cycle, one follicle on the ovary will grow sufficiently to release an egg into the Fallopian tube. But with polycystic ovaries, many follicles will develop, not reaching full mature size but creating clusters of follicles on the ovary.

Symptoms of PCOS include:

- irregular periods
- no periods
- irregular or no ovulation
- excess hair on the face, breasts or insides of the legs
- acne
- oily skin
- lack of sex drive
- mood swings and/or depression
- weight gain and difficulty losing weight despite efforts to do so
- food cravings

PCOS doesn't affect all sufferers with fertility problems, but it is certainly a concern, and it may also be a factor in women who experience recurrent miscarriages.

Often PCOS causes the ovaries to go haywire, as they start to produce hormones in incorrect proportions. Too much testosterone influences hair growth, while oestrogen dominance can affect the luteal phase (see page 168). Luteinizing hormone (LH) may go out of balance, affecting ovulation. If high levels of insulin are produced, this may stimulate the ovary to overproduce testosterone and prevent the follicles from growing normally to release eggs.

Treatments
- The contraceptive pill is often offered to help regulate the cycle, although this is by artificial means and so doesn't treat the cause. It's important to still have a good diet and lifestyle.
- Metformin may be prescribed to control insulin resistance, which may be the cause for PCOS in some women. This drug re-sensitizes the body to insulin, in turn encouraging the ovaries to produce a more healthy balance of hormones. It can help to induce ovulation and may help to control the inflammation in

the body caused by PCOS. You may be prescribed a combination of metformin and statins if PCOS has caused your cholesterol level to rise.

- You may also be offered surgery, especially if you are undergoing assisted reproductive treatment (see page 206).

Toolbox

Drugs may give you a temporary rebalancing effect for your hormones but there are also many things you can do through diet and lifestyle that will have the same effect – and last. There are three things to consider: emotional issues, diet and erratic lifestyle.

Mind and PCOS

Frustration, irritability and depression are all signs that the Qi energy of the body, and in particular the Liver, is Stagnant and congested, which may then affect the release of an egg. Feelings of anguish or anxiety particularly affect the Heart, which can also delay ovulation.

If you are conscious of these emotional states being an issue for you, the chapter on Fertility Mindfulness (see page 116), should help you to gain awareness of how your emotions and ovulation can influence each other.

Diet

Diet can play a big role in PCOS, which is often associated with being overweight or having too much Damp in the body (feeling puffy or bloated with excess water). This is made worse by eating too many sweet, greasy or dairy foods, irregular eating habits, too much alcohol and drinking on an empty stomach. Dr Marilyn Glenville's book *Natural Solutions to PCOS* (see Resources) gives a full nutrition plan. Here are some tips for you to try:

- Switch to unrefined carbohydrates. While I am a big fan of white rice in moderation for most people, as it is very easy on the digestion, in the case of PCOS white rice is best avoided, as are white pasta and bread.
- Eat regularly to keep your blood sugar levels balanced.
- Eat plenty of omega-3 fats, including oily fish and flax seeds.
- Cut down on saturated fats, and avoid all trans fats.
- Avoid alcohol to support your liver.

- Eat plenty of green leafy and cruciferous vegetables to support the liver and balance your hormones.
- If you are showing signs of excess testosterone (excess hair growth), cut out dairy for three months to see if this helps.
- Cut down on caffeine.
- Losing weight can be difficult with PCOS as it is a metabolic-related disorder. I am a fan of following the low-GI diet, as it is very much tailored to addressing insulin resistance in a healthy way (see Resources).

Lifestyle

- Stress only makes PCOS worse, so it's a good idea to practise the ways of calming the mind I have described throughout the book (see Stress on page 26 and Fertility Mindfulness on page 116).
- Be aware of hormone disruptors in your environment (see page 28).
- Research suggests that acupuncture and exercise improve the symptoms of PCOS.[61, 62]

FIBROIDS

Fibroids are benign tumours found in the uterus. They are thought to affect up to 40 per cent of women, but most often women will not experience any symptoms and the fibroids won't affect fertility. They occur more frequently in women of Afro-Caribbean descent, and also in women who have not had children or are overweight (fibroids are linked to oestrogen and overweight women often have oestrogen dominance).

Fewer than one in three women experience symptoms of fibroids, which may include heavy periods, pain during intercourse, infertility, urinary or bowel problems. Fibroids can cause problems if you do become pregnant, and they can become bigger during pregnancy, so they will be closely monitored if detected.

Where the fibroids are situated can make quite a difference to how they affect you. Submucosal and intramural fibroids are more likely to cause painful or heavy periods, as well as problems with implantation of an embryo or miscarriage. Subserosal and pedunculated fibroids are more likely to cause pain, especially during pregnancy.

Treatments

There is still quite a bit of debate over if and when to treat fibroids, as it is unclear whether they really do affect fertility and chances of conception. One thing doctors agree on is that when fibroids are causing great discomfort, treatment should be seriously considered.

- For older women who aren't looking to get pregnant, hormonal treatment is often the best approach. For younger women, submucosal fibroids can often be treated by a hysteroscopy (see page 250), alongside a gonadotropin-releasing hormone analogue (as used in IVF) which decreases oestrogen levels, causing the fibroids to shrink so that removal is easier.
- A myomectomy may also be used; this is the name of the surgical procedure to remove fibroids. An incision is made along the bikini line, and great care must be taken to repair the muscle to reduce the risk of adhesions (see page 17). If a myomectomy is performed and you later become pregnant, a Caesarean section will usually be advised to protect against possible rupturing of the uterus.
- As a last resort, a hysterectomy may be needed for very severe fibroids, but only in cases where the fibroids are so large and the uterus has become so distorted that pregnancy would not have been possible.

Toolbox

- Help to regulate your hormones (which may contribute to the fibroid growth) through a high-fibre, low-GI diet (see Resources).
- Include plenty of omega-3 fatty acids in your diet by eating oily fish and flax seeds.
- Support your liver to balance your hormones by eating leafy greens, cruciferous vegetables (cabbages and broccoli) and fermented foods like sauerkraut and pickled cabbage (see page 97).
- Maintaining a healthy weight is important (see page 56).
- Be aware of your environment and cut out xenoestrogens when you can (see page 28).
- Exercise regularly to help balance your hormones (see page 102).

- I give acupuncture to help move the Blood, as fibroids are a sign of Blood Stagnation. It is particularly important to have acupuncture during the period itself and in a month when you know you are not pregnant, from ovulation onwards.

THYROID PROBLEMS: HYPOTHYROIDISM

Thyroid problems are often overlooked and yet they can be the missing link for women with unexplained infertility, especially in the case of hypothyroidism (underactive thyroid).[63] Every cell in our bodies depends on the thyroid hormones for regulation of metabolism, energy production, weight maintenance and use of oxygen.

Hypothyroidism can affect fertility in the following ways:

- disrupting ovulation
- shortening the luteal phase (see page 184)
- oestrogen dominance
- progesterone deficiency

As we have seen in other chapters, these are some of the main causes of fertility problems, so addressing any thyroid problems can be the key for some women. It can be hard to spot them, though, as the symptoms tend to differ from person to person. Commonly reported symptoms of hypothyroidism include:

- exhaustion
- weight gain
- dryness of hair, nails and skin
- loss of libido
- sensitivity to cold and difficulty getting warm (check whether your BBT is consistently lower than 36.5°C/97.7°F)
- mood swings
- poor memory
- constipation
- menstrual irregularities
- period pains
- recurrent infections

Treatment

You can be treated with drug hormone replacers, but this is often a lifelong therapy. Making changes in your own diet, lifestyle and environment can make a real difference.

Toolbox

- Developing ways to calm the mind is very worthwhile as stress is thought to be a major factor in all hormone-related conditions, including hypothyroidism.
- Exercise is beneficial as helps to stimulate thyroid hormone release.
- Limit your exposure to chemicals and heavy metals and try to maintain a healthy environment (see page 28).
- Watch out for any foods you may be allergic or intolerant to. Wheat is a big culprit for many people, and wine can cause problems due to the sulphates.
- Support your digestion with a relaxed but healthy diet (see page 62).

THYROID PROBLEMS: HYPERTHYROIDISM

Hyperthyroidism (overactive thyroid) can affect fertility by disrupting your menstrual cycle, leading to irregular or a lack of periods. This is turn can affect ovulation. Common symptoms and signs of an overactive thyroid include:

- hyperactivity
- mood swings
- insomnia
- tired all the time
- feeling weak
- sensitivity to heat and excess sweating
- unexplained weight loss
- need to pass urine or stools often
- irregular periods
- irregular or fast heart rate
- tremor or shake/twitch
- warm moist and/or red skin/excess sweating

- itchy skin
- swelling in neck (enlarged thyroid gland)

Treatment

Your doctor will refer you to an endocrinologist (a specialist in hormonal conditions), who may offer the following:

- Thionamides: these stop the thyroid being overactive.
- Beta-blockers: may be prescribed to help with specific symptoms such as shakes or tremors.
- Radioiodine: a form of radiotherapy that shrinks the thyroid in one dose. Women are advised to avoid getting pregnant for six months following this treatment.
- Surgery is rare and usually reserved for recurrent cases.

Toolbox

- Selenium and vitamins B6, B2 and B3 are helpful for hormone balancing.
- A healthy diet is helpful (see page 62) and include foods with plenty of essential fatty acids like oily fish, avocado, nuts and seeds.
- Clean up your environment – use natural products where possible.
- If you have thyroid antibodies, take steps to lead a more balanced lifestyle and have treatments such as acupuncture.

MISCARRIAGE

Sadly, I have seen many women experience miscarriage and I myself have had two. It's not something that people talk about much; but I think there is now more openness about this painful experience, and you may be amazed at how many people are willing to share their stories as a form of support when the subject is broached.

Why do miscarriages occur?

About half of all fertilized embryos never implant or do not implant well enough to develop into a pregnancy. Sometimes a woman may sense she was briefly pregnant or may even get an early positive pregnancy test, but then it fails to progress.

The causes of miscarriage are not easy to establish. Possible causes include: a problem with a pregnancy, which causes the body to reject it; hormonal imbalances; problems with the sperm, uterus, implantation, placenta, cervix or immune system; or an infection of some kind. The most common reason for a pregnancy failing is because the embryo has a chromosomal abnormality, such as Trisomy 21, which causes Down's syndrome. These abnormalities are more common in older women, and so the miscarriage rate is higher as you get older. The extremes of BMI are also associated with an increased risk of miscarriage, both in natural pregnancies and after fertility treatment.[64]

ECTOPIC PREGNANCY

An ectopic pregnancy occurs when the fertilized egg implants outside the womb. This usually occurs in one of the Fallopian tubes, or less commonly in an ovary, the cervix or the abdominal space. The pregnancy can't be saved; but early diagnosis and treatment improves the chances of being able to experience a normal pregnancy at a later date.

After a miscarriage

Following a miscarriage, it's essential to establish that all placental products have been discharged. In some cases a sharp curettage may be needed to make sure the uterus is free of all the tissue that needs to be expelled. This small operation is performed under general anaesthetic.

Most of the work I do around miscarriage involves helping women recover, as well as helping women who have had miscarriages in the past with subsequent pregnancies. Research suggests that when women are well supported in subsequent pregnancies following miscarriage, it can improve pregnancy outcome.

Like so many aspects of female fertility, the Qi and the Blood are an important consideration following a miscarriage, particularly if there has been heavy loss of blood. Follow the guidelines for nourishing the Qi and the Blood (see pages 81 and 65) and make sure you take adequate time to recover. Raspberry leaf tea is an excellent tonic, as is nettle tea. Aubergines help to move the Blood and have a strong tonifying effect on the uterus.

In terms of the emotions, my experience is that some women will want to 'get back to normal' as quickly as possible. For many this approach works just fine; they are happier getting on with their life and do not feel the need to dwell on the sadness and the loss. If this applies to you, just make sure it is really how you are feeling and that you are not just acting that way for everyone else's benefit. Others may find it much harder to recover; I have met women who are haunted by the loss for many years. Do give yourself some emotional and physical time out. Your body will have been pumped full of pregnancy hormones and the drop in these is bound to contribute to feelings of sadness.

Men too suffer during a miscarriage, as they also experience the emotions of loss. Clearly they do not go through the physical process of losing a longed-for baby, but emotionally it can be hard for them, and difficult for them to know how to help. It's hard when your partner is sad and difficult to console, but there is no need to suffer in silence.

When to start trying again

The temptation is sometimes to have another baby as soon as possible to replace the loss, and that can work out well for some couples. It really depends on the nature of the miscarriage. My first miscarriage was very early, at seven weeks, and I conceived my second daughter the following month. However, my second miscarriage came much later in the pregnancy and I was quite unwell, having suffered from a significant loss of blood, and had to stay in hospital for several days. After that experience, I made the decision not to put myself through it again. My view was that I had two daughters and I was already blessed. It's up to the individual; no one can judge the right way to respond. Had I decided to have another go after the second miscarriage, I think I would have needed at least four months to get over it physically (and emotionally it can take longer). Of course age is a consideration, but even so it is usually better to enter a subsequent pregnancy in good health than to rush into it too soon.

SECONDARY INFERTILITY

Secondary infertility is the inability to become pregnant following one or more successful pregnancies. One in seven couples struggle with secondary infertility, and many of the patients I see at my clinic are finding it difficult to conceive a second or third child. Even for couples who conceive relatively easily the first time, it can sometimes take a long time to conceive another baby.

It can be emotionally difficult when you desperately want another child and you are unable to understand why things are taking longer. Many women report that they find it hard to be with friends who have managed to conceive again, as they feel inadequate and desperate for another baby. There is also often little sympathy extended to women in this situation, as they are perceived to be lucky to have any children at all.

Sometimes it is simply a matter of reduced opportunity: it can be hard to fit in sex when you already have one or two children and you are tired from broken nights. Furthermore, there is a growing trend to have our children in quick succession with very little gap in between. We see other couples achieve this and assume it is the norm. In previous generations, when child-rearing was spread out over a much longer time frame, it was quite normal to have large gaps between children. My own mother had five children spread over a twenty-year period. I like to think of this as 'organic parenting': my parents used no contraception and sometimes they tried to avoid pregnancy by avoiding the fertile times, but the rest of the time they just 'got on with it' (according to my mother).

Interestingly, according to Chinese medicine, a woman ideally needs five years between children to recover her energies and to make space in order to give proper care and attention to the next child. With the average age of a woman having her first child being twenty-nine, this would be impossible for most families, and it has become necessary to have children much closer together.

So how do you know if you have a problem, or whether it is normal or simply lack of opportunity? As a general guide, if you are having regular sex (every two or three days throughout the month) and you have not conceived within a year, you should seek help. Research suggests that couples who have had one or more children and are seeking fertility treatment are more successful and have more live births than couples who have had no previous pregnancies.

It is important to consider the following factors:

- Have your periods returned to normal?
- Did you breastfeed for longer than nine months? This can result in the Blood becoming Deficient. Acupuncture and herbal medicine can help.

- Have you gained or lost a significant amount of weight? If so, you might need to get your thyroid tested.
- Weight can also affect conception if your BMI is too high or too low (see page 39). Make sure you maintain a healthy weight and eat a healthy diet.
- Did you lose a lot of blood in the delivery or afterwards? Again, this can result in Blood deficiency.
- Did you have retained products of birth which were hard to pass or that had to be surgically removed? You might need a scan to check that the uterine lining is clear and there are no adhesions (see Asherman's syndrome, page 17). A scan can also check for fibroids and infections that can develop after childbirth. Problems of this kind can often go undiagnosed, and they are usually very treatable.
- Did you have a traumatic birth or suffer from postnatal depression? If the answer to either question is yes, you may need to work through this with a counsellor. I am a big believer that sometimes our mind can block our body from achieving pregnancy, particularly if you have experienced trauma.
- It is worth your partner getting a sperm test. Sometimes sperm problems can develop, particularly if your partner has had an acute illness with a fever.
- It's important to remember that as you get older your fertility does naturally reduce, so while age may not have been a factor in your first pregnancy, it may play a part if it takes longer to get pregnant again.

I'd really encourage you to resist the habit of comparing yourself to other people. We are all different; just because those around you are having babies close together, that doesn't mean you have to follow suit. Do what is right for you and your family and also what is right for your body.

CHAPTER ELEVEN
ASSISTED REPRODUCTION

Although there is a big part of me that wants to believe nature is always best or superior, I know that some couples who would make wonderful parents will need the helping hand of medical intervention to have a baby. A major part of what I do is to support couples through fertility treatment. I play the role of giving the patient some fine-tuning with acupuncture, helping the body to function optimally, helping to create a calm mind, and listening to what they say and what they don't say (often what they don't say is an indication of where they may benefit from help). The diet, mindfulness and lifestyle advice I give in this chapter will sound familiar, as I am again looking to nourish the Blood, calm the mind and warm the Womb.

Every year more couples seek help from assisted reproductive technologies (ART). In 2010 just over 45,000 women had IVF treatment in the UK and nearly 58,000 cycles were undertaken, with 12,714 babies born as a result.

The ICSI technique (see page 230), which involves choosing sperm to inject into the egg, now counts for 52 per cent of fertility treatment in the UK, and egg freezing is growing in popularity. As yet, there isn't a treatment that can promise to overcome the challenges of age. These are the current statistics for successful fertility treatment in this country, broken down by age:

under 35:   32.3 per cent
35–37:   27.2 per cent
38–39:   19.2 per cent

40–42:   12.7 per cent
43–44:   5.1 per cent
45+:   1.5 per cent[65]

Approximately one in seven couples have difficulties with fertility. The main factors for men are either low quality or volume of sperm; for women age is the main factor, alongside damage to the Fallopian tubes (see page 21), problems with ovulation (see page 172) and endometriosis (see page 191). In a third of cases the cause is never established, which is why I also pay such close attention to the roles of mind and lifestyle when it comes to fertility, as well as being aware of menstrual, gynaecological and sexual health. I really believe that older patients need to take more control of their general lifestyle and that healthy living becomes paramount. There is also a growing body of research to indicate that acupuncture can improve the chances of successful embryo transfer and also of live birth. My role is to support patients through this process, both physically and also by helping them to support themselves emotionally and with nourishing food. Becoming a mother through what can feel like a very clinical process is all about keeping in touch with the bigger picture. IVF can be a difficult journey, and taking time to look after yourself, getting more rest and supporting yourself with things like acupuncture can really be of benefit.

If you do seek support from complementary medicine while undergoing any fertility treatment, always talk to your specialist or consultant about this. It is widely accepted as a helpful support by the Western medical community, and it is very useful for them to know about all your treatment. And I do encourage you to follow the general advice in this book while you are waiting for treatment, as getting your body healthy for conception and pregnancy is extremely worthwhile, whatever path your fertility journey may take.

WHEN TO SEE YOUR GP

The vast majority of couples conceive naturally within a couple of years, but you don't need to wait that long to have a chat with your GP. They might initially encourage you to keep trying and get as healthy as possible for conception and pregnancy. They will also want to establish whether there are any underlying conditions that may be affecting your fertility and that you don't yet know about, like PCOS (see page 194) for example. If you suffer from a fertility-related condition, the priority might be to address that first, although this might depend on other factors like age.

The next step might include a number of basic tests:

- cervical smear test
- urine test to check for chlamydia (which can cause blocked tubes)
- blood tests before and during your period to check that ovulation is occurring and also for possible hormone imbalances (FSH, LH and oestradiol)
- sperm test (see page 45)

If these tests reveal any fertility issues, or if after a time there is still no clue as to why you might be struggling to conceive, you will probably be referred to a fertility clinic to see a specialist. Further investigatory tests include:

- full hormone profile during your period
- AMH test (see page 32)
- ultrasound scan of the uterus and ovaries
- follicle tracking: a series of scans following the development of a follicle to check if and how the egg develops
- hysterosalpingogram (see page 250): an X-ray of the Fallopian tubes
- laparoscopy (see page 193) to check for any blockages in the Fallopian tubes
- hysteroscopy: using a camera to check inside the womb for fibroids or polyps
- hysterosalpingo-contrast sonography (HyCoSy): checking for blockages using an ultrasound probe
- endometrium lining tissue sample testing

FERTILITY TREATMENT OPTIONS

It seems like there are new breakthroughs in fertility treatment reported in the papers almost daily. Getting to know what's really available and what might be right for you as an individual can be quite a minefield. I've enlisted the help of the consultants and specialists I work with to ensure I've included all the current options. I'll also go through the IVF process in detail, along with ways you can support yourself during the cycle.

Common fertility drugs
Clomifene citrate (Clomid)
How it is taken: In pill form.
What it is for: To stimulate and/or regulate ovulation.
Possible side effects: Hot flushes, mood swings, nausea, breast tenderness, insomnia, increased urination, heavy periods, spots, weight gain. May also slightly increase risk of ovarian cancer if taken for over a year.

Personally, I think this drug works very well for some but can be detrimental to others. It does stimulate the ovaries but at a cost to the Yin and Blood, so if you are Deficient in these areas to begin with, it may not be the best approach.

Metformin
How it is taken: In pill form.
What it is for: Used in the treatment of PCOS to stimulate ovulation.
Possible side effects: Nausea, vomiting, diarrhoea, abdominal pain, metallic taste, itching, allergic reactions and, in rare cases, hepatitis.

Follicle-stimulating hormone (FSH); Puregon luteinizing hormone (LH)
How it is taken: Injections (one per day). When eggs are mature, you are given an injection of human chorionic gonadotropin (hCG) hormone to trigger release of an egg (or eggs).
What is it for: Stimulates the ovaries to produce eggs. Can be used to treat PCOS in cases in which Clomid hasn't worked. Also used to treat infertility due to pituitary gland failure and some male infertility.
Possible side effects: Overstimulation of the ovaries (see page 225), risk of multiple pregnancy when used for ovulation induction, allergic reactions and skin reactions.

Drugs to regulate your treatment cycle
During treatment, your doctor will usually prescribe other drugs for you to take at various times to give more control over your treatment cycle. These may include the following:

Gonadotropin-releasing hormone (GnRH)
How it is taken: Nasal spray, several times daily, or as daily injections or monthly depo (injected under the skin) before, or at the same time as, taking fertility drugs.

What it is for: To stop the natural menstrual cycle.

Possible side effects: Hot flushes, night sweats, headaches, vaginal dryness, mood swings, changes in breast size, breakouts of spots, acne and sore muscles.

Gonadotropin-releasing hormone antagonists

How it is taken: Daily subcutaneous (under the skin) injection. Given at the same time as FSH injections.

What it is for: To stop ovulation until eggs are ready to be collected as part of the IVF cycle.

Possible side effects: Nausea, headaches, injection-site reactions, dizziness and malaise.

Progesterone

How it is taken: As a vaginal suppository, a pill, gel or by injection into the buttock, either after the injection of the pregnancy hormone hCG, or on the day embryos are returned to the womb. I know some clinics have a preference for the injection method, and I have noticed this seems to give good results, although it is rather an unpleasant injection.

What it is for: To thicken the lining of the womb in preparation for nurturing a possible embryo after IVF or IUI.

Possible side effects: Nausea, vomiting, swollen breasts.

Bromocriptine and cabergoline

How it is taken: In pill form.

What is it for: Reduces high levels of prolactin hormone, which can interfere with production of and the effect of FSH.

Possible side effects: Nausea, headache, constipation, dry mouth, skin reactions, hair loss, lowering of the voice.

What is intrauterine insemination (IUI) and how does it work?

Intrauterine insemination (IUI) is a procedure in which fast-moving sperm are separated from slow or non-moving sperm. The sperm with better motility are then placed into the woman's womb close to the time of ovulation.

Your clinic may recommend IUI for the following:

- unexplained infertility
- ovulation problems

- male partner experiences impotence or premature ejaculation
- trying for a baby using donated sperm.

It is essential to make sure that your Fallopian tubes are known to be open and healthy before the IUI process begins. This is usually assessed by your clinic using a laparoscopy and dye test (see page 193) or a hysterosalpingogram (see page 250). When the pelvis and tubes are healthy, dye passes freely through both tubes. It is also important to check that there is no significant issue with sperm numbers or sperm quality.

IUI TOOLBOX

Remember to support IUI in the same way as you would your menstrual cycle (see page 159). So at the start of the cycle look to nourish the Blood and Yin, and concentrate on building follicles. Many women have acupuncture as a support prior to and post IUI treatment.

How does IUI work?

For women:

Step 1: The procedure will usually take place between day 12 and day 16 of your monthly cycle (counting day 1 as the first day of your period). Blood or urine tests will identify when you are about to ovulate and many clinics will provide you with an ovulation testing kit to detect the hormone surge that signals imminent ovulation.

Vaginal ultrasound scans track the development of your eggs and as soon as an egg is mature, you will be given a hormone injection to stimulate its release. If you are taking Clomid, look out for excess Heat in your system and balance this by introducing some cooling foods and teas like rosebud or camomile (see page 247).

Step 2: The sperm are inserted 36 to 40 hours later. The doctor inserts a speculum into your vagina, as in a cervical smear test. A small catheter (a soft, flexible tube) is then threaded into your womb via your cervix and the best-quality sperm are selected and inserted through the catheter.

The procedure takes just a few minutes and is usually painless, though some women may experience a temporary, menstrual-like cramping. Meditation can be helpful at this point as a way of switching the brain off. Try to be as relaxed as possible, as a calm mind helps release an egg smoothly.

Step 3: You may feel you need to rest for a little while before going home. Ask your clinic what they recommend.

For men:
Step 1: You will need to produce a sperm sample on the day the treatment takes place.

Step 2: The sperm are washed to remove the fluid surrounding them and the fastest moving sperm are separated out.

Step 3: The separated sperm are placed in a small catheter (tube) to be inserted into the womb.

What is in vitro fertilization (IVF) and how does it work?

In vitro fertilization (IVF) literally means 'fertilization in glass' – hence the term 'test-tube baby'. During IVF, eggs are removed from the ovaries and fertilized with sperm in the laboratory. A fertilized egg (embryo) is later placed back in the woman's womb. One in eighty babies born in the UK is now conceived through IVF.

Your clinic may recommend IVF as your best treatment option if:

- you have been diagnosed with unexplained infertility
- your Fallopian tubes are blocked
- other fertility treatments, such as fertility drugs or IUI (see page 210), have been unsuccessful
- there is a minor degree of male subfertility (more severe problems are treated with intra-cytoplasmic sperm injection (ICSI))

How does IVF work?

IVF techniques can differ from clinic to clinic, but typically the procedure will involve the following steps:

For women:

Step 1: Suppressing the natural monthly hormone cycle

As the first step of the IVF process, you may be given a drug to suppress your natural cycle. The most commonly used drug is a gonadotropin-releasing hormone agonist (GnRH agonist). Treatment is given either as a daily injection (normally self-administered, unless you are not able to do this yourself) or as a nasal spray. Sometimes this treatment starts about a week before menstruation in the cycle before you start stimulation, and will continue for about two weeks before you start stimulation. This is known as the long protocol, and it is becoming less popular. Some clinics prefer to start the GnRH agonist on day 1 of your cycle, at the same time as you start the FSH injections. This is known as the short or flare protocol.

Many doctors now use a GnRH antagonist, which is given by injection starting after about six days of FSH stimulation. This is more easily tolerated by most and more convenient, but the number of eggs collected (or egg yield) is slightly lower. This is not important for most women, but it can be critical in those who are termed 'poor responders' (see page 218).

I normally treat women once a week with acupuncture for a week or two before their treatment cycle starts. The purpose at this stage is to improve liver function and calm the mind.

Step 2: Stimulation phase

This is achieved by daily injections of FSH, lasting for around 12 days. This hormone will increase the number of eggs you produce, meaning that more eggs can be fertilized. With more fertilized eggs, there is a greater choice of embryos to use in your treatment.

The work to begin building a good endometrium also starts during this phase. It is important to get adequate protein and Blood-nourishing foods (see page 65) and enough rest. I see women twice a week during this phase and use acupuncture to help pelvic Blood flow and to encourage the follicles to grow evenly on both sides by increasing Blood flow to the slower side.

Step 3: Monitoring progress

The clinic will use vaginal ultrasound scans and, possibly, blood tests to monitor your progress throughout the drug treatment.

Around 34–38 hours before your eggs are due for collection, you will be given a hormone injection to help the eggs mature.

Step 4: Egg collection

Eggs are usually collected under sedation by ultrasound guidance. A needle is inserted into the scanning probe and into each ovary. The eggs are then collected through the needle. Cramping and a small amount of vaginal bleeding can be experienced afterwards.

If you have had a difficult collection in the past, I suggest acupuncture the day before to help relax the patient, as well as the ovaries and reproductive area in general. Acupuncture in between egg collection and transfer is a great opportunity to improve Blood flow, relieve any bloating and generally work on making the body more receptive and calming the mind.

Step 5: Fertilizing the eggs

Your eggs are mixed with your partner's (or the donor's) sperm and cultured in the laboratory for 24 hours, before checking to see how many have fertilized normally.

These embryos are grown in the laboratory incubator for another one or two days before being checked again to make sure they are growing normally. Usually, the best of the embryos are transferred back to the uterus on day 3 or if you have enough good embryos, they will be cultured for another two days until they reach the blastocyst stage on day 5. This is a hollow ball of cells; the inner cell mass (ICM) will form the foetus and outer cells (trophectoderm) will become the placenta. The best one or two embryos will then be chosen for transfer. Reflexology is helpful at this time.

After egg collection, you are given progesterone to help prepare the lining of the womb for embryo transfer either in pessary form, an injection or gel.

During this time, it is good to focus on becoming receptive: eat warming foods, keep warm and stay calm. I use acupuncture to help return the body to normal function and establish a healthy Blood flow. If ovarian hyperstimulation syndrome (OHSS) is suspected (see page 225), acupuncture can be very helpful to ease bloating and drain fluids from the abdomen. I have seen women walk into my clinic with bloated abdomens, only to walk out after their treatment fitting comfortably back into their jeans.

Step 6: Embryo transfer

For women under the age of 40, one or two embryos can be transferred. If you are 40 or over, a maximum of three embryos can be used. There is a maximum because of the risks associated with multiple births (see page 226). Remaining embryos can be frozen for future IVF cycles.

I don't advocate rushing around immediately before and after embryo transfer or getting stressed by too many appointments, including acupuncture sessions. I prefer to see patients in the days after the transfer to aid implantation and calm the mind during the two-week wait to find out whether implantation has been successful. There is research to suggest that acupuncture can be helpful at this time, but I liken this limited use to putting a seed in the soil and then adding fertilizer at the last minute. For me, the key is in the preparation of the soil and the seed.

For men:

Step 1: Collecting the sperm

Around the time your partner's eggs are collected, you will be asked to produce a fresh sperm sample.

Step 2: Selecting the best-quality sperm

This sperm is stored for a short time and then washed and spun at a high speed to select the healthiest sperm.

If donated sperm is being used, it is removed from frozen storage, thawed and prepared in the same way.

Natural IVF

With this technique minimal or no medication is used, so you will usually produce only one or two eggs per cycle. The success rates are lower (5–8 per cent), but avoiding drugs can be better for some women and may allow them to conceive in a natural cycle. When thinking about fertility preservation and preserving women's health in the long term it's important to consider natural or 'mild' IVF as an option. For some women this is a good alternative to using higher doses of stimulation to the ovaries. Combined with therapies such as acupuncture and supported by good nutrition, I believe mild IVF could be a better approach for some couples.

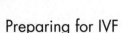

Preparing for IVF

Below I have listed some complementary treatments you might want to try prior to starting IVF. It's not necessary to use all of them; perhaps pick a few that appeal to you and can be undertaken easily. I don't want you to feel you have to run around doing every treatment, causing yourself more stress. After these treatments I have included other factors, like weight management, that are all worth considering too.

Many women suffer from congestion or Stagnation in the pelvic cavity and reproductive system, especially with conditions such as endometriosis, PCOS and previous surgery, including Caesarian sections. Women who lead a very sedentary lifestyle can also suffer from congestion in the reproductive system. Make sure you keep active without overdoing it, getting too hot or sweating too much.

Acupuncture

As you might expect, this is my first choice of therapy to use as preparation and support through IVF. Acupuncture has such a regulating effect on the body, gently improving pelvic Blood flow, improving the endometrium and moving any Stagnation in the pelvic region. Studies have shown that the increased blood flow improves the number of follicles that will respond to the stimulation drugs.[66] It is also deeply relaxing and helps the patient prepare mentally for IVF. Weekly acupuncture for six weeks prior to starting IVF is ideal.

Acupuncturists are frequently asked by patients to reduce their FSH levels; by doing this we are not able to improve the quality of the eggs, but I do believe we are able to affect the function of the ovaries. It is important to address all aspects of the patient's health.

Around implantation, acupuncture is used to help increase Blood flow and the flow of Qi to the endometrium and pelvic cavity to improve receptivity.

Manual lymphatic drainage

The lymphatic system is a vast network of capillaries and nodes that removes and destroys toxins, transports nutrients and hormones throughout the body and eliminates excess fluid from the tissues. Manual lymphatic drainage (MLD) is a gentle, repetitive form of massage that encourages fluids to move more freely around the body. In the month prior to starting IVF a couple of MLD treatments can be very helpful, especially for women who have had several cycles of IVF.

Herbal medicine

At my clinic we often use herbal medicine in preparation for IVF. My colleague Kate Freemantle says: 'Through my research and clinical experience I have seen women who have previously had a poor response to IVF and low AMH become pregnant after taking Chinese herbal medicine. A recent meta-analysis study has suggested that management of female infertility with Chinese herbal medicine can improve pregnancy rates two-fold within a four-month period compared with Western medical fertility drug therapy or IVF.[67]

'However, this is not a quick fix. Herbal medicine needs to be taken daily for a period of three to six months. My belief is that this time frame could be important due to the three months (or more) that it takes for follicles to develop.'

Colonic irrigation

Having colonic irrigation prior to IVF may help to decongest the pelvic cavity and generally help the flow of Blood and energy in the area. I think it is worth including, especially for women who have been through several cycles of IVF. Do not have more than a couple of treatments, as they can deplete the system if performed too often.

Colonic irrigation may also be helpful for immune system and implantation issues, as it helps the gut to function better and will reduce inflammation. If the gut is functioning well, it helps remove excess oestrogen from the body, which if left in the bowel for too long gets reabsorbed back into the Blood stream in its unhealthy form.

Weight management

Any weight-loss programme should be started several months before commencing IVF. It is not recommended to lose weight too quickly. I always advocate eating regularly, and advise patients not to be tempted to go for low-fat foods as natural, full-fat foods are better for embryo production and quality. See page 56 for advice on healthy weight loss.

Poor responders

This is a term applied to women who produce few eggs during IVF or eggs of poor quality. I hate this terminology and prefer to talk about Yin Deficiency or Blood Deficiency. The quality of the egg is affected by ovarian function, age, general health, constitution and lifestyle. My main advice here is to really take it easy, get plenty of rest and nourish yourself well. Avoid harsh detox diets, build up your energy reserves, meditate, get early nights, eat regular meals, avoid coffee and try not to burn the candle at both ends. Generally take good care of yourself.

FSH

Most clinics require that women have an FSH of 10 or under (an indicator of your ovarian responsiveness; see page 32) to be considered for IVF. In truth, the only absolute way of knowing how a woman will respond to IVF is by going through the process. I have had many women with unfavourable hormone levels respond quite well to treatment and go on to have healthy babies. In my own practice, I see FSH as an indicator of how hard the ovaries will have to work to produce follicles, and this gives me an idea of how much support and preparation is needed. I use FSH as just one of many tools to assess a woman's fertility and never make a judgment based on FSH (or AMH) alone.

CoEnzyme Q10 and DHEA

Some clinics advise taking CoEnzyme Q10 and/or DHEA to help improve egg production and embryo quality (see page 35).

Whey protein

Some clinics ask patients to drink large amounts of milk during IVF to help embryo quality, but I prefer to recommend whey protein. Take one scoop in a glass of water mixed with raspberries and half a teaspoon of cinnamon three times a week in the month prior to IVF, and then every day during the stimulation phase of the cycle.

Endometrial scratch

One other recent addition to fertility treatment has been the use of endometrial scratching. This simple procedure, performed in the month before an IVF cycle, stimulates the lining of the uterus. It can be undertaken as a separate procedure (a little like an embryo transfer), or as part of a formal assessment of

FOLLICLE BOOSTING IVF PROTEIN SHAKE

Blend the following:

> *protein powder (follow instructions on the packet)*
> *2 handfuls of raspberries*
> *1 teaspoon of flax seeds*
> *1 cup of water or nut milk*

- Drink three times a week in the month prior to IVF and every day during the stimulation phase of the IVF cycle.
- Drink first thing or as a mid-morning snack.
- If you are trying to avoid dairy or are intolerant, replace with another high protein powder like pea and hemp/rice protein (see Resources).

the uterus at a hysteroscopy. According to consultant gynaecologist Michael Dooley (see Resources), it is believed that scratching the lining of the womb causes a reaction that releases growth factors and other chemicals. This may make the womb more likely to accept an embryo.[68]

Implantation issues

Once the egg has been fertilized by the sperm to create an embryo, that does not guarantee implantation or that ultimately pregnancy will occur. While Western medicine tends to focus on collecting good-quality eggs, implantation is of equal importance, as this is the point at which so many pregnancies fail, particularly IVF pregnancies. It is likely that this will be due to both embryo and endometrium issues.

Of course, genetically abnormal embryos are likely to make up a large proportion of those embryos that fail to implant, particularly when a couple are in their late thirties or forties. However, it is important to consider other potentially treatable causes. These may include lack of (or inhibited) Blood flow as a result of trauma, repeated miscarriage or Asherman's syndrome (see page 17). Hereditary blood-clotting disorders (such as Factor V Leiden) may also impact on implantation.

This is an area in which I feel acupuncturists have a great deal to offer women. I have seen on many occasions how acupuncture has been able to improve endometrium thickness and receptivity. In many ways, helping the system to function optimally and thereby improving the receptivity of the body is what acupuncturists have done for time immemorial. However, acupuncture is not a miracle cure, and the results will very much depend on the individual and the reasons behind the implantation failure.

I find that assessing the menstrual bleed and taking a full medical history is a good way of establishing if pregnancies are failing at implantation stage.

Medical treatments for implantation issues
IVIG
Intravenous immunoglobulin is a blood product made from human blood plasma. It is used as an immune suppressant by some fertility clinics to reduce natural killer (NK) cell activity and aid implantation.

Humira
This is another immune suppressant drug (used to treat rheumatoid arthritis), which is used by some private fertility clinics on women who have had recurrent implantation failure and in cases where immune-system issues are suspected.

Blood thinners
Heparin and aspirin are increasingly used during IVF to thin the blood and aid implantation. The evidence supporting the use of these drugs is not clear, but I have seen women achieve successful implantation when using them.

Cinnamon is a natural blood thinner, which is why I suggest taking it during IVF (see my IVF smoothie on page 219). If you are taking a blood thinner such as heparin or aspirin, don't have more than a very small amount of cinnamon.

Reproductive immunology
Many advances in reproductive technologies have been made in Western medicine, particularly in the area of IVF. However, most of it has been focused around selecting the strongest-looking embryos, and there have been relatively few advances in the area of implantation. There are several theories in circulation regarding the role the immune system might play in implantation. Treatments aimed at suppressing the immune system and

reducing the level of natural killer cells are on the increase, but without sufficient scientific research to back up their efficacy, these approaches remain in the realm of private medicine.

Some years ago, when Dr Alan Beer (the author of *Is Your Body Baby Friendly?*; see Resources) was alive, I was lucky enough to sit in on some of his consultations regarding reproductive immunology. This is the idea that sometimes pregnancies fail at implantation due to issues with the immune system. One of the questions I asked him was which group of women should be considered for immune testing. His view was that this procedure should be offered to women who had repeated IVF failure despite good embryo quality; women with autoimmune conditions or a strong family tendency to autoimmune conditions (such as rheumatoid arthritis, Crohn's disease and thyroid antibodies); women with endometriosis; and women who have had abnormal embryos implant.

Although reproductive immunology is still quite controversial I believe there are women for whom this may be the central issue. The role of the immune system is often underplayed or ignored. Interestingly, when I first studied Chinese medicine twenty years ago, a Chinese doctor said to me: 'You will see that the immune system has a huge role to play and we will see it affecting all sorts of areas of health, including fertility. Now we see a great deal of deficiencies in the immune system, but the immune system is also capable of being overactive as well.' How true his words turned out to be, and how strange that this was to become such a big part of how I practise today.[69]

EMOTIONAL PREPARATION

You will know very well by now how much importance I place on a calm mind. Being stressed and having high levels of cortisol (the hormone secreted by stress) can reduce progesterone and cause your body to create too much oestrogen. It is important to reduce inflammation in the body and increase serotonin. Read the chapter on Fertility Mindfulness again and try any of the following to help you feel relaxed and positive: acupuncture; massage; counselling; meditation; yoga; and spending time with people you love and care about.

The IVF mind
Before starting IVF, everyone worries about injecting the drugs, but actually the drugs can be quite a good distraction from the really hard aspect of IVF:

the mind. Emotionally, IVF treatment can be a roller coaster. For a start, your hormone levels are being manipulated; but also you will need to steel yourself to get through each stage successfully.

Of course, for many, starting the treatment can be exciting, especially after going through months of the frustration of not conceiving and wondering why. Everyone deals with it differently, but it can be hard getting through each stage. The two-week wait to find out if the embryo has implanted is especially challenging. It's important to remain as philosophical about it as possible, as you cannot change the outcome. Although some patients convince themselves it hasn't worked, my experience is they are often wrong, so it's important to keep the faith.

How to stay strong and focused during IVF

There is so much to worry about in IVF:

- Will I produce embryos?
- Will my partner produce a sperm sample?
- Will the sperm fertilize the egg?
- Will the embryo make it to blastocyst stage?
- How will I cope with the two-week wait?

The most important thing to remember is that children are born through the union of your relationship. Of course children are also born under all sorts of circumstances, but if you are going through IVF with a partner, remember that you are both in it together.

Do little things to support one another. Some men may have to put up with listening to constant talk of babies and IVF, even if they aren't that interested in all the detail. And women also need to learn to try to switch off from the subject. Men and women process things in different ways; some women process stuff by talking it over – and over and over! Often men deal with things by only engaging in what they absolutely have to. I don't want to get too stereotypical here, but in my experience about 90 per cent of couples do fall into certain roles in this situation.

I think a lot of men don't know what to do to help, and most women don't want to have to expend energy explaining what it is they need. Of course, some couples find that they easily support one another in the right way and instinctively know what each other needs. This is wonderful and they are blessed; don't ever lose that, as it is a precious thing. Other couples have different dynamics and have different reasons for being together. Many spiritual beliefs maintain that we choose our partners so that we can learn from them the lessons we need to learn in life. A relationship is like a mirror being held up to us, constantly reinforcing the part of our personality or psyche that needs attention. Going through huge life-changing experiences gives us each an opportunity to learn and grow. It's hard to view IVF and the infertility struggle in this way; I do not mean to underplay the intensely emotional challenges it presents to couples. But it does give you a chance to deepen your experience of life with each other.

IVF STORE CUPBOARD

Below are some suggestions of things to stock up on before starting IVF, so that you always have some nutritious foods to hand.

- Dark green leafy vegetables (for example, spinach, kale, watercress) help to support liver function. Buy organic if possible.
- Dandelion tea is good to help a congested liver; it also improves digestion. Nettle tea is good for the Blood.
- Green tea contains catechins which help protect the liver.
- Essential fatty acids: eating oily fish is also good for the liver.
- A plentiful supply of nuts and seeds is good for snacks as they are high in protein and healthy fats.
- Beans, soya and lentils are all high in protein, as is tofu.
- A good supply of chicken stock, homemade if possible (you can prepare a batch in advance and freeze it).
- Chlorella, spirulina and whey protein are all good sources of protein, essential for the production of embryos.
- Oily fish such as mackerel.
- Seasonal foods and herbs.
- You will need to drink plenty of water: try to buy in bulk, but avoid plastic bottles in favour of glass.

Congee

Congee is simply rice cooked slowly in much larger quantities of water than we are often used to. The rice is cooked until it breaks down and turns the liquid thick and creamy. Congee has a mild, sweet flavour and is incredibly easy on the digestion, so it is very nourishing and healing. (For those with PCOS, who benefit from a low-GI diet, brown rather than white rice is advised.)

Congee is a mild dish, so it's the perfect base for other flavours, from warm stewed fruit in the morning to fresh ginger, chicken and sesame oil as a nourishing evening meal.

How to prepare congee

Rinse one cup of plain, polished short-, medium- or long-grain white rice (not basmati) and add to a heavy-bottomed saucepan along with 5–10 cups of water (5 cups will give you more of a 'sticky rice' consistency; 10 cups will be quite soupy). If you are making savoury congee, you might want to add some chicken or vegetable stock for a nice flavour.

Bring the rice to an easy boil and then reduce to a low simmer for between 30 and 90 minutes, depending on the consistency you prefer. Stir occasionally to prevent the rice sticking to the bottom of the pan.

The longer you can wait the better.

During the stimulation phase of IVF, eating some chicken or egg congee would be ideal. After the embryo has been transferred, add warming spices and try a sweet ginger version. If you are in the post-transfer stage and you feel overheated and agitated, try the cooling congee (see below).

Chicken congee: Prepare the congee with chicken broth or stock. Stir-fry chicken in sesame oil and serve with the congee in individual bowls, along with thin slices of fresh ginger and spring onions.

Egg congee: Prepare your basic congee with water or chicken stock. Five minutes before serving, crack one egg per person on top of the congee and allow to set before serving. Season with sea salt and black pepper.

Sweet congee: Prepare your congee with a few slices of fresh ginger. A few minutes before the end of cooking, add some slices of fruit (or stewed fruit), a little honey and a dusting of cinnamon.

Cooling congee: Prepare the congee with coconut milk added to the water. Serve with fresh pineapple and banana.

CAN I HAVE SEX DURING IVF TREATMENT?

Many couples abstain from sex during IVF for various reasons: lack of time; stress; being more focused on the medical treatment; or because they fear an orgasm may dislodge an embryo. Many clinics advise abstaining from sex. However, some studies have suggested that the presence of semen in the vagina after embryo transfer is likely to have a positive impact on implantation after IVF, perhaps due to its effects on the female immune system. Sex after embryo transfer may not be advisable for women with OHSS and/or any abdominal pain or distension.

RISKS OF FERTILITY TREATMENT

Ovarian hyperstimulation syndrome (OHSS)

OHSS is a side effect of the stimulation drugs given during an IVF cycle, and it will occur in around 1 per cent of cycles. In these rare cases, the ovaries become abnormally enlarged and develop large cysts, which produce fluid that is then released into the abdomen. Symptoms include abdominal pain and swelling, shortness of breath, nausea, possible vomiting, and a lack of urine. In severe cases (0.25 per cent) hospitalization may be necessary to replace fluids, minerals and protein and to prevent further complications.

As with just about all medical conditions, prevention is better than cure. I always advise my patients to be aware of whether they are developing a strong thirst and/or dry mouth. Women with PCOS (see page 194) are thought to be at a higher risk of OHSS. And patients who respond particularly well to the stimulating drugs and produce lots of eggs may also be at greater risk, particularly if they experience abdominal pain before egg collection. If this is the case, the treatment cycle may be cancelled, or the embryos may be frozen to give time for things to settle down, so preventing OHSS symptoms from becoming more serious.

Remember that OHSS can progress if a pregnancy is achieved, especially a twin pregnancy, as there are twice as many hormones.

Tips to prevent OHSS

- If you are high risk, ask to be scanned as early as day 5 after embryo transfer.
- Drink plenty of water.
- Eat a high-protein diet to help to metabolize the IVF drugs.
- Call your clinic straight away at the first sign of symptoms, as catching this early can help a great deal in the long run.
- See an acupuncturist. I have seen that this can make all the difference.

Multiple births

According to the HFEA, having a multiple birth (twins, triplets or more) is the single greatest health risk associated with fertility treatment. According to research, the risk of losing a child before birth or within the first week of life is more than four times greater for twins than for a single baby. The risk of cerebral palsy is five times higher for twins, and eighteen times higher for triplets. If you choose the option of single embryo transfer, the risks are greatly reduced, so it is worth talking through the pros and cons with your own consultant.

Single embryo transfer

At the embryo transfer stage, couples are sometimes given the choice between transferring one or two embryos. Couples understandably want to increase their chances of becoming pregnant, so transferring two embryos can seem appealing; also there is the chance of having two babies at once and not having to go through IVF again.

Blastocyst transfers (see below) have reduced the need to transfer more than one embryo in most cases. Transferring two blastocysts means that you have a success rate of 60 per cent, and a 50 per cent chance of having twins. With a single blastocyst transfer, the success rate is 55 per cent.

There are of course cases where it is appropriate to transfer two embryos, such as day 3 transfers in older women, or for women who have previously gone through a failed cycle. Make sure you talk it through with your consultant early on in the process, so that you are prepared when it comes to making the decision. From my understanding of energy, I don't always think 'more is more'; some women seem to fare better from a single embryo being transferred.

One of the issues is the complications that can occur with multiple pregnancies. It is also important to consider that a single embryo can split and become two, so potentially two embryos can become triplets. I have seen this happen on quite a few occasions and sadly it does not always have a happy ending.

Embryo reduction is sometimes offered to some women with multiple pregnancies when the situation is considered a danger to mother or child. For some women there is no choice if they are to stand a chance of carrying even one baby to term. Patients must wait until 12 weeks to select the embryo for reduction, to avoid terminating a healthy baby in favour of a genetically abnormal one. Couples will need proper information to help them decide to transfer one or two embryos. Always discuss this fully with your consultant and embryologist.[70] More information is available at the Human Fertilization and Embryology Authority website (see Resources).

Blastocyst transfer

Most clinics now offer blastocyst transfer, a procedure in which the fertilized eggs are left to mature for five to six days; the developed embryo is known as a blastocyst. After egg collection, the eggs and the sperm are put together in order for fertilization to occur. The transfer takes place around the day-5 stage of development of the embryo; not all embryos will make it to this stage.

Blastocyst transfer is used when there are a good number of embryos, as it allows the embryologist to determine which embryo is best for transfer into the woman. Getting a good number of blastocysts is associated with an increased likelihood of pregnancy. The other advantage with the procedure is that it allows clinics to choose just one embryo to transfer, reducing the risk of multiple births.

If there are not a high number of embryos (this will differ from clinic to clinic and will be determined by the embryologist), the embryos are likely to be transferred at day 3. Although couples may feel disappointed when this happens, it is important to remember that there may still be a pregnancy as a result. In fact, I have had several patients who have done both day-3 transfers and blastocyst transfers and have only been successful with day-3 transfers.

Interestingly, the first three days of development of the embryo are under the maternal influence; it is only after three days that the paternal influence kicks in. So if you find your embryos are making it to three days and then declining in quality or ceasing to develop, you may want to look at ways to improve male fertility. Speak to your clinic and take a look at The Fertile Man chapter on page 42.

FROZEN EMBRYO TRANSFER – IS FRESH ALWAYS BEST?

During the course of an IVF cycle, embryos are sometimes left over. If they are of good enough quality, these can be frozen and implanted back into the mother at a later date. Historically, these frozen embryos have been considered less likely to go on to implant successfully, as some of the quality is lost during the freezing process.

So far, most evidence suggests that fresh gives better results. However, there is some early evidence to suggest that, with freezing methods improving all the time, frozen embryo transfers may be more appropriate in some situations, using a process known as vitrification (which is also used for freezing immature eggs; see page 34). A study done at Aberdeen University found that babies born as a result of frozen embryo transfer were less likely to be premature or underweight and the mother was less likely to experience bleeding during pregnancy.[71]

However, a practical consideration standing in the way of more frozen embryo transfer is NHS-funded IVF. Many clinics will only provide one fresh cycle and will not include a frozen one. This is unfortunate as women are more likely to opt to put more than one embryo back which is not necessarily ideal and may well lead to more problematic pregnancies (see Single Embryo Transfer on page 226). Although most IVF units still say, 'fresh is always best', I have felt for some time that in certain patients transferring embryos back immediately after strong stimulation to the ovaries may not always be the best thing to do. Some women respond quite strongly to the stimulation drugs and can become extremely bloated and their ovaries very enlarged. I also think that leaving time between stimulation and implantation can give the endometrium time to recover, particularly if supported with acupuncture.

Certainly, in terms of energy, I find that some patients fare better than others during IVF. I feel that some of them could benefit from a period of time when the system is returned to normal function and a good Blood flow established to the endometrium to help make it more receptive.

In the following cases, patients may benefit from a frozen embryo transfer:

- **Male factor IVF:** Increasingly, couples are going through IVF due to male factors, when there is no known problem in the woman. Many of these women will be under thirty and therefore likely to respond very well to the stimulation drugs. Clinics should be aware of this and should stimulate the woman very gently, so as to avoid overstimulation. In this case, freezing the embryos to transfer at a later date may well have benefits.
- **Ovarian hyperstimulation syndrome (OHSS):** If a woman has developed this condition (see page 225) and she becomes pregnant during that cycle, the condition can continue and even worsen as the body is flooded with pregnancy hormones. There may well be an argument for freezing the embryos to transfer later.
- **Implantation issues:** There may be a case for using frozen embryos when implantation issues are suspected, as the period between collecting embryos and transferring them into the womb could be extended, giving an opportunity to prepare the woman for transfer. Preparation could include the methods described on page 220, or by using acupuncture, herbal medicine and other natural methods.
- **High levels of progesterone:** The presence of too much progesterone during an IVF cycle has been associated with poor outcomes and severely reduced success rates. Freezing the embryos and waiting for a cycle when the progesterone

has reduced to a level less than 5 is advisable. It is not clear why, though it's possible the endometrium may be stimulated by progesterone too early on in the cycle.

- **Endometriosis:** Theoretically the endometrium may benefit from a period of time after the stimulation phase, so that it has a chance to rest and recover.
- **Hydrosalpinx:** When there is fluid present in the tubes and/or uterus, it may be deemed necessary to delay transfer.

These ideas are based on my own clinical experience and my understanding of how the body's energies respond to IVF stimulation. More research needs to be done in this area to establish which patients could benefit the most. The dilemma will always be the trade-off between embryo quality and patient receptivity. Until such a time when we can demonstrate which patients (if any) will benefit, I suspect that most clinics will stick to the notion that 'fresh is best'.

Intracytoplasmic sperm injection (ICSI)

Last year more than 23,000 intracytoplasmic sperm injection (or ICSI) treatments were performed. ICSI is a procedure used during IVF to treat male subfertility. A single sperm is injected directly into an egg, and then the egg is left to develop before being transferred into the uterus.

Intracytoplasmic morphologically selected sperm injection (IMSI) is a form of ICSI in which higher magnification is used to choose the sperm. There is some debate as to whether or not this advance is a positive one. It takes longer and so that might be an argument against it, as the egg will only be viable for so long, but if it means better sperm are chosen, the outcomes may be better in the long term. There isn't enough research to support a firm conclusion at present.

A piece of research was published recently which threw up some potentially worrying statistics about ICSI and birth defects. According to the *New England Journal of Medicine*, researchers from the University of Adelaide in Australia looked at more than 300,000 births and found that one in ten babies born through ICSI suffered some form of birth defect. In naturally conceived babies the proportion was one in twenty. They found that babies born via ICSI were 57 per cent more likely to suffer some form of abnormality.[72]

However, when I spoke to James Nicopoullos at the Lister Fertility Clinic about this, he described his own position, which is based more on the huge meta-analysis that came out at the same time as the Australian study:[73]

'The Australian study actually included around 6,000 ART [assisted reproductive technology] births, whereas Wen et al looked at 125,000 babies born through ART. They did confirm what consultants are already very aware of: that babies born through ART have a higher birth defect risk (37 per cent increase), but the study raised three important questions. The first was whether this showed a true rise. Many of the studies that looked at defects do not take into account maternal age, twin rate, duration of fertility and other factors that play a role. Even those couples who had fertility issues but conceived naturally also had a significantly increased risk of birth defects (54 per cent), so it may be that there is something intrinsic in these couples themselves that increases the risk rather than the treatment itself. The second question was whether ICSI was really worse than IVF. It turned out that the Wen meta-analysis included 24 studies that directly compared IVF and ICSI (46,980 IVF and 27,754 ICSI), with no difference in the birth defect rate between the two.

'The third question was how to quantify the actual rise in risk. If you take the recent Europe-wide paediatric EUROCAT study that showed a 25.4/1,000 risk of birth defects and factor in a 37 per cent increase for IVF/ICSI babies, then 34.5/1,000 ART babies will have a birth defect. So the risk goes up from 2.5 per cent to 3.4 per cent, which is probably not going to really stop someone who needs IVF or ICSI from doing it.

'The only time that I am concerned about ICSI is when a man has a severely poor [sperm] sample and hasn't had a karyotype/Y deletion test. Even if that is normal, he may have a slightly higher proportion of sperm that are aneuploid [having an abnormal number of chromosomes], which we don't routinely check, and this is why perhaps ICSI babies have a slightly higher risk of subtle genetic abnormalities that haven't obviously been passed on.'

IVF OR ICSI?

- **IVF:** Egg(s) and sperm are put together in the petri dish and the embryologist waits for spontaneous fertilization to take place.
- **ICSI:** The embryologist selects one sperm which is injected into the egg.

ICSI has been the most significant advance for male subfertility in the past three decades. Although first used in cases of poor sperm motility, it is far more widely used now. There is some debate as to whether using ICSI for all may improve IVF outcomes. Until now it has been mostly used to improve IVF outcomes in cases of male subfertility or when fertilisation rates have been very low in previous cycles.[74, 75]

Donor insemination (DI)

In this procedure, the sperm of a known or anonymous donor is placed inside the woman's uterus using a syringe. This is the best option for single women and lesbian couples. It is also an option to consider when the male partner is sterile or is a carrier of an inherited disease, or when IVF has failed.

Egg donation

This is an option for women who are unable to produce their own eggs. It is never an option taken lightly, but can represent a couple's best chance of carrying a baby. Egg-sharing schemes are run by some IVF clinics; the eggs will come from women who are undergoing IVF due to male-factor infertility. Your partner's sperm will be used to fertilize the egg before being transferred to your womb.

Gamete intrafallopian transfer (GIFT)

As with IVF, this technique is used to stimulate the ovaries and collect eggs. The best eggs are mixed with the sperm, and then both are transferred to the woman's Fallopian tubes for fertilization to take place. It is a technique used occasionally in cases where there is unexplained infertility, problems with the cervical mucus (see page 153) or mild endometriosis (see page 191). However, there is an increased rate of multiple births, with the associated risks, and a laparoscopy is also necessary to transfer the embryos. Very few clinics offer GIFT now.

In vitro maturation (IVM)

In this procedure, eggs are removed from the ovaries and collected when they are still immature. They are then matured in the laboratory before being fertilized. This means that the woman does not need to take as many drugs before the eggs can be collected as she might during conventional IVF, when mature eggs are collected. However, it is really only useful for women with PCOS, who may have a large number of immature follicles.

Surgery

Some minor fertility problems can be addressed and treated during a laparoscopy (see page 193). Microsurgery, using a microscope and very small instruments, can also be an option.

Surgery may be used for the following conditions:

- adhesions or blockages to the Fallopian tubes or ovaries
- endometriosis (see page 193 for all treatments)
- a narrow or scarred cervix
- fibroids (see page 197)
- an abnormally shaped uterus
- sterilization reversal
- ovarian cysts and endometrial polyps

Pre-surgery tips
- Check with your doctor to find out if you need to stop taking any medications, including any complementary nutrition or herbal supplements.
- Stock up your cupboards and freezer with nutritious foods that are easy to prepare; see recipes for congee (page 223) and chicken soup (page 72).
- Give yourself time to heal properly after the surgery before trying to conceive.
- Get friends and family to be on standby to help.

- Concentrate on maintaining a healthy lifestyle pre-surgery, so reduce your workload and stress, drink little or no alcohol, eat well and get plenty of rest.
- To aid with healing, for one week before surgery take the following supplements: vitamin C, 2,000mg once a day; bromelain digestive enzymes, 500mg three times a day between meals; arnica, 2 30c tablets placed under the tongue three times a day.

Post-surgery tips

- Be aware that your body will be tired during the healing process, so plenty of rest is crucial.
- Eat lots of nutritious food.
- Keep alcohol to a minimum during the recovery period.
- According to Dr Adrian Lower, patients may find the following complementary remedy helpful: Pycnogenol (a natural anti-inflammatory and antioxidant), 60mg twice a day.
- Keep taking the vitamin C, bromelain and arnica supplements (see Pre-Surgery Tips above) for one week after surgery.
- Start taking vitamin E one week after surgery to aid healing and reduce scar formation.
- Acupuncture is recommended after surgery to restore good Blood flow.

CONCLUSION

The documentary *March of the Penguins* is the story of a remarkable fertility journey of one species. Each year, as they have done for millennia, the Emperor penguins leave the comfort of the sea to walk single file over the ice to their traditional breeding grounds, enduring blinding blizzards, to meet, court and mate with a lifelong partner.

The creation of life is a miracle in all species. The emperor penguin endures immense hardship in order to ensure the survival of its species. They are driven by instinct, a deep drive within them: a determination to continue to survive in the harsh terrain that is their home, where no other living creature can survive, let alone breed. They are quietly heroic in their mission – it is a mission of love.

These are qualities I see in clinic every day: the immense, deep, unwavering drive to have a child. Sometimes it is forgotten that people can suffer deeply if their instinct to reproduce is thwarted. We are all creatures of this earth, and to conceive offspring is one of the greatest urges we have, even if it is often unspoken. I have huge admiration for these women and men who go through so much in order to have their longed-for child. Theirs is a silent, heroic quest. Often their suffering is not understood by others, who may think that because these people are not ill, they do not suffer.

Humans will always strive to reproduce, and many will go to the ends of the earth in order to achieve their goal. Most will eventually be successful, even in the most unlikely and inhospitable of conditions when it may seem that all hope is lost. I have seen many couples who, like the penguins, continue to keep faith and persevere. It has always been thus; we will continue to live out our own reproductive ritual for time immemorial. It is our story of love: love against all odds.

AFTERWORD

This book was written for, and will no doubt be read by, women and couples who want to be pregnant NOW. But within its pages is an important wider message: the idea of fertility and health preservation. It is never too late to improve your health and fertility, but to what extent this is possible is harder to answer. We are putting off parenting until later in life, and technology is advancing all the time. With that has come the expectation that if we want to have a baby in our forties, it ought to be possible.

Health preservation is central to how I practise; the way we look after ourselves and how we live will impact on the quality of our health for our whole life. Much of Western medicine is not based on this principle; it does not encourage us to nurture and engage in our health in quite the same way. Instead, there is an unspoken promise that the professionals will take care of us when things go wrong. With that comes a willingness to hand our health over to others. Surely it is better to take some responsibility ourselves – to take what steps we can to preserve our health and our fertility. When we do engage in our health, we become happier and healthier more quickly.

Women today belong to the 'you can have it all' generation. Why should we have it all? 'Because we're worth it.' I think we all know that turned out not to be true for so many. We grew up knowing not to take drugs because we would end up a crumpled mess like the guy in the anti-drugs poster, and we got the message that unprotected sex can lead to AIDS. There were no cautionary tales about our fertility waning with age. The only advice women were given about babies was to wait, enjoy ourselves and have a career first. The teenage mum was our cautionary tale.

I was lucky enough to have a mother who told me that we children (all five of us) were the biggest achievements of her life. It was a good message; but many women, myself included, want more than that.

I have had women – intelligent women with great jobs and lives – come into my treatment room and say things like 'Nobody told us it might be too late' and 'I had no idea my fertility would take such a dip in my late thirties.'

Many working environments are not baby-friendly for women. For men who work in the City, children are seen as a status symbol, showing the fathers to be steady and reliable. But for a woman in the City, a baby can be seen as a setback. We all look much younger than our mother's generation, and we have many youth-enhancing, age-defying treatments and potions at our disposal. But this does not stop our eggs from ageing – we cannot Botox our ovaries!

Of course, age is by no means the only factor affecting fertility. Not all women are equal: we will all age at a different rate, and many women will be able to have babies into their forties (while many young women will struggle to conceive, without knowing why). Can we slow down the ageing process? I believe we can, a little, and perhaps even rejuvenate our fertility – a little.

When I meet a new patient, these are questions I constantly find myself pondering:

- What are the factors that are impacting on their fertility?
- Can we do anything in the future to prevent or limit the damage?

More research is needed into the ovarian environment. For many years we have been too focused on the egg and the sperm. But the environment in which the egg develops is vital, and this may well prove to be the one area that we *can* affect. Equally, the womb, which will play host to the baby for nine months, must be in optimal condition. Men, too, must take their role seriously and learn to nurture good health prior to conception so as to preserve their fertility. It is never too late to take steps to improve your health, and I hope that this book will encourage you to do so.

So my hope is this: that the next generation will look to us and learn – learn that fertility is precious and needs preserving.

When you have finished reading this book, please give it to a younger woman in your life.

WHAT I TELL MY PATIENTS

Fertility awareness
Protecting your fertility
- Learn about STDs and protect yourself.
- Avoid perfumed feminine-hygiene products.
- Learn how to drink alcohol responsibly.

Preserving your fertility
- Get to know your Jing (constitution); don't compare yourself to others.
- Ask your mum: your mother can help you understand your physical and emotional inheritance.

Lifestyle
Diet
- Stick to natural, unprocessed foods, don't eat anything blue except blueberries.
- Don't count calories or obsess about your body.
- Aim to be neither overweight nor underweight. For good health, average body weight really is best.
- Swap coffee for herbal teas; eat chicken soup.

Exercise
- Listen to your body for when you need to move Stagnation and when you need to restore Qi (energy).
- Always take the stairs.
- Remember the importance of rest. Nothing good happens after midnight.

Friends
- Surround yourself with positive people.
- Avoid people who see the world through a negative haze.
- Surround yourself with your own interior strength.

Environment

- Reduce toxins in your environment.
- Try to find natural approaches to manage minor health conditions.
- Illness can be a great teacher: learn what makes you ill and make changes accordingly.

Mind

- Know yourself and be true to yourself.
- Strive for balance.
- When we heal ourselves, it has repercussions for our world.
- Learn to say no. Emotional truth is a much undervalued virtue.
- Be positive and have gratitude for all the gifts in your life.
- Value your intuition: listen to the quiet voice inside yourself.
- Love is our true nature.

Menstrual cycle awareness

- Engage in your menstrual cycle and gynaecology: it is a wise woman's guide.
- Being a woman is an awesome thing, and your periods are all part of that.

Sex

- Women's sexuality is about giving and receiving sexual pleasure, as well as the instinct to reproduce.
- Remember that it is your choice who you have sex with and when.
- Have the courage to understand your needs and what gives you pleasure.

Male fertility

- Protect your testicles from heat and injury.
- Protect yourself from STDs.
- Address any health issues before they become chronic.

Fertility-related conditions

- Don't become a Google addict: seek professional advice rather than looking up symptoms online.

- Stay on top of your gynaecology in your twenties and thirties.
- Seek help following miscarriage or childbirth if you don't recover your former health.

My best advice for ART

- Seek help if you have been having regular sex for a year and have not conceived.
- Make a plan. Research well and spend time choosing the right people.
- Try acupuncture to help optimize your fertility.
- Strike a balance between being informed and becoming obsessive. It's a hard one.

APPENDIX I
FERTILITY TOOLBOX: BASIC TREATMENT PRINCIPLES

Qi Stagnation
Signs
- irritable bowel syndrome (IBS)
- premenstrual syndrome (PMS)
- pelvic inflammatory disease (PID)
- sighing and frowning a lot
- feeling irritable
- prone to mood swings, tears and anger
- indecisiveness
- struggling to finish projects and move on
- feeling uncomfortable in your body
- mauve tinge to the tongue
- feeling uncomfortable and bloated after eating
- swollen breasts
- irregular periods
- tenderness under the ribs
- struggling to feel balanced and positive
- sleep affected by frustrations
- feeling stuck and frustrated

Toolbox
- Try clearing out a messy cupboard or sorting out your wardrobe. Don't try and do too much, just enjoy the feeling.
- Change your behaviour habits to help get out of a rut, like taking a different route to work or going for a walk at lunchtime.
- Don't dwell on issues too much. Get on with something useful to distract yourself and keep yourself moving.
- The feeling of completing a project is just what those suffering from Qi Stagnation need.

- Watch or do something that will really make you laugh.
- Get some physical exercise: a brisk walk, swimming, dancing, any kind of sport.
- Look after your liver and cut down on alcohol.
- Eat light Qi-supporting foods (see page 81).
- Beware of comfort eating.

Blood Stagnation

Signs

- pain at the site of surgery
- broken veins and capillaries under the skin
- varicose veins
- fibroids
- endometriosis
- feeling tired and heavy
- stabbing pains
- bruising easily
- extremities easily getting cold
- pins and needles
- purple tongue and purple hue around the mouth
- swollen veins under the tongue
- purple dots along the tongue
- stabbing pain and blood clots at the start of your period

Toolbox

- Eat Blood-moving foods such as aubergines (see page 65 for a full list).
- Try abdominal massage.
- Drink spiced citrus tea: mix the juice of half a lemon, a teaspoon of grated ginger and half a teaspoon of cinnamon into a mug of hot water.
- See a gynaecologist to check for any underlying conditions.
- I often recommend seeing a Chinese herbalist in conjunction with acupuncture and orthodox treatments (see Resources).

Blood Deficiency
Signs
- scant menstrual flow or amenorrhoea (no periods; see page 162)
- pale complexion
- dull, dry skin
- dry hair
- pale lips and tongue
- dry and brittle nails
- orange tinge on the sides of the tongue
- dizziness
- seeing spots in front of your eyes (floaters)
- forgetfulness
- overworking
- difficulty falling asleep
- feeling unsettled in bed
- feeling of anxiety, sometimes with a rising panic in your chest
- prone to panic attacks
- restless mind
- easily startled
- slim build
- prone to catching any bugs going around

Toolbox
- Eat plenty of blood-nourishing foods (see page 65).
- Eat regular meals in a relaxed environment.
- Eat lots of leafy greens and sesame seeds.
- Black or deep-red foods are good, as is seaweed.
- Eat plenty of protein.
- Cut out alcohol.
- Cut out sugar.
- See a Chinese herbalist (see Resources).
- Try to maintain a good work–life balance.
- Don't over-exercise.

Damp
Signs
- allergies such as asthma or hay fever
- skin conditions like eczema

- oily complexion
- candida or thrush
- thick cervical mucus
- mucus in stools
- foul-smelling stools
- overweight or slim but with cellulite
- preferring to be sedentary
- crashing out when you fall asleep
- legs feeling heavy
- feeling bloated after eating
- finding it difficult to concentrate
- fuzzy head

Toolbox

- Avoid alcohol (especially beer), dairy foods (especially cheese), chocolate, curries (especially if you also experience signs of Heat), bread, wheat, sugar and fried foods.
- Don't drink too much water.
- Don't eat late at night.
- Don't eat protein at the same time as carbohydrates like grains – stick to protein with vegetables or grains with vegetables.
- Eat lots of bitter leaves like watercress, onions, garlic, aduki beans, alfalfa sprouts, celery, chicory and fennel.
- Drink jasmine tea, green tea and fennel tea.
- Include herbs and spices in your diet, such as cardamom, ginger, sage, thyme and parsley.

Cold
Signs

- abdomen is cold to the touch
- water retention
- needing to urinate frequently, and producing a lot of clear urine
- loose bowel movements
- taking time to get things finished
- taking a while to build enthusiasm
- white coating on tongue
- pale complexion

- sluggish digestion
- prone to putting on weight easily
- medium to low libido
- preferring to stay in with a good book and a hot-water bottle
- feeling worse in cold weather
- sleeping deeply
- finding yourself often sitting near or even on the radiator

Toolbox

- Drink warming teas such as ginger and sweet chai (see page 88).
- Eat warming foods like soups, stews, carrots and squash.
- Keep warm with blankets and plenty of layers.
- Take baths with essential oils such as bergamot, orange, cardamom and cinnamon.
- Sleep well away from any draughts.
- Practise yoga stretches.

Heat

Signs

- often very thirsty, needing to have water by the bed
- throwing off the covers during the night
- feeling charged and energetic
- feeling frustrated, restless or agitated
- red in face
- strong-smelling sweat
- red tongue
- yellow coating on tongue
- finding it difficult to relax
- feeling constant hunger and tending to binge

Toolbox

- Avoid caffeine, tobacco, alcohol, chocolate, greasy foods, sugar and stimulants.
- Develop ways to calm your mind (see page 26).
- Practise meditation.
- Practise yoga.

APPENDIX II
FERTILITY GLOSSARY

adhesions – Scar tissues that attach to the surfaces of organs.

AMH – Blood test that measures the level of anti-Müllerian hormone (AMH), a hormone that is released by your ovaries. This can be used to estimate a woman's ovarian reserve (egg supply) to give an indication of how much longer they will be fertile.

andrologist – Specialist in men's reproductive issues.

anovulation – Absense of ovulation (menstruation may still occur).

anti-phospholipid antibodies (APLAs) – Proteins that may be present in the blood and may increase your risk of blood clots or pregnancy losses.

anti-nuclear antibodies – Antibodies that target 'normal' proteins within the nucleus of a cell.

anti-sperm antibodies – Antibodies that attack the sperm cells; these can be produced by both men and women.

antral follicle count – Used to predict a woman's IVF success rate and her likely response to ovarian stimulation.

Asherman's syndrome – Scarring in the uterus, usually from a previous procedure, for example a sharp curettage (scraping) following miscarriage or to remove the placenta after giving birth, a Caesarean section or surgery to remove fibroids or polyps.

aspirin – May be prescribed alongside IVF to improve chances of conceiving.

assisted hatching – A microinjection procedure which chemically dissolves the embryo surface to facilitate implantation.

azoospermia – Absence of sperm in the seminal fluid, which might be due to a blockage or an impairment of sperm production.

basal body temperature – Your body temperature taken as soon as you awake. Recorded daily, this can help determine when and if ovulation is taking place during your cycle.

beta-hCG test (BhCG) – Blood test to detect pregnancy.

biochemical pregnancy (also chemical pregnancy) – Positive hCG level in the blood that doesn't continue to rise and so does not lead to pregnancy.

blastocyst – Fertilized egg developed for five or six days (until this time described as an embryo).

blighted ovum (egg) – An egg that is fertilized but fails to implant/survive in the uterus.

bromocriptine (Parlodel) – Medication used to lower prolactin levels.

cancelled cycle – Discontinuation of the IVF cycle due to either poor response, no egg recovery or failed fertilization.

cervical mucus – Secretions produced by the cervix which vary in quantity and consistency throughout the month.

Clexane – Drug used to stop blood clots forming.

clomifene (Clomid) – Drug used to stimulate production of FSH and LH, often used to treat women who are not ovulating.

cultures – Tests for infections in men and women.

ectopic pregnancy – When the fertilized egg implants outside of the uterus, usually in the Fallopian tube, ovary or abdominal cavity.

egg donation – When eggs are removed from one woman to be used by another.

egg freezing – When a woman's eggs are collected and frozen for future use.

embryo freezing – When embryos are frozen during the IVF process, either for potential future use or to give time for the body to prepare for implantation.

endometriosis – Presence of uterine lining in areas outside of the uterus, including the Fallopian tubes, ovaries and bowel.

endocrine disruptors – Man-made chemicals that can interfere with normal hormonal function.

endometrium – Mucus membrane lining the uterus.

ERPC – Evacuation of retained products of conception.

Fallopian tube – Transports the eggs from the ovary to the uterus. This is where fertilization usually takes place.

fibroid – Non-cancerous tumour in the uterus.

foetal reduction – Procedure in assisted reproduction to decrease the number of foetuses in a multiple pregnancy.

follicle – Fluid-filled sac on the ovary, from which the egg is released at ovulation or collected during an IVF cycle.

follicle-stimulating hormone (FSH) – Hormone produced in the anterior pituitary gland that stimulate the ovary to grow a follicle.

FSH test – Test used to assess ovarian reserve.

follicular phase – Phase of the menstrual cycle during which follicles develop (after a period, pre-ovulation).

genetic screening (IVF) – Analysis of chromosomes for abnormalities in the IVF process.

gonadotropin – Hormone that stimulates the testicles to produce sperm and the ovary to produce an egg.

hysterosalpingogram (HSG) – X-ray of the Fallopian tubes and uterus, done seven, eight or nine days before ovulation.

Humira – Drug used to treat immune system conditions.

hysteroscopy – Used to investigate potential causes of very heavy or irregular menstrual bleeding, and in some cases to treat scarring (for example, Asherman's or endometriosis).

intra-cytoplasmic sperm injection (ICSI) – Injection of a single sperm directly into an egg in order to fertilize it. The fertilized egg (embryo) is then transferred to the woman's womb.

Intralipid – Fat emulsion that has been shown to lower the activity of NK (natural killer) cells.

intrauterine insemination (IUI) – Procedure to separate fast-moving sperm from more sluggish or non-moving sperm, which are then placed into the woman's womb close to the time of ovulation.

in vitro fertilization (IVF) – Procedure by which eggs are removed from the ovaries and fertilized with sperm in a laboratory. The fertilized egg (embryo) is later placed in the woman's womb.

laparoscopy – Surgical procedure used to investigate and treat some gynaecological conditions.

lupus – Immune-system illness, probably genetic in origin and mainly affecting females.

luteinizing hormone (LH) – Hormone produced by the anterior pituitary gland which causes the egg to be released by the ovary and stimulates progesterone production. In the male, LH stimulates testosterone production.

luteal phase – Phase in the menstrual cycle after ovulation and before the period starts.

male factor infertility, male subfertility – When a couple's fertility problems are attributed to male factors.

metformin – Used in the treatment of PCOS to stimulate ovulation.

molar pregnancy – An unsuccessful pregnancy in which the placenta and foetus do not form properly and a baby does not develop.

motility – Percentage of moving sperm in a semen sample.

MTHFR – Genetic abnormality in clotting, indicated in some miscarriages. Treated with high doses of folic acid and aspirin to thin the blood.

natural killer (NK) cells – Immune-system cells that normally help the body fight infections. There is now an idea that in some women these cells may attack the foetus as though it is an invader. It is a contentious area, but some doctors do advise using drugs to suppress the action of NK cells.

oestrogen – Female hormones produced by the ovaries.

oligospermia – Low sperm count.

oocyte – Egg produced by the ovaries (also: ovum, gamete).

ovarian cysts – Small fluid-filled sacs that grow on the ovaries.

ovarian drilling – A surgical treatment that can trigger ovulation in women with polycystic ovary syndrome (PCOS).

ovarian hyperstimulation syndrome (OHSS) – Possible side effect of IVF, when ovulation is medically stimulated, resulting in swollen, painful ovaries and sometimes bloating from fluid retention in the abdomen or chest.

ovarian reserve – The age or health of the ovaries and the eggs they contain.

oxidative stress – A physiological stress caused by the body's inability to adapt to free radicals. It is the most accepted theory for premature ageing and is also indicated in a number of diseases, including cancer, Parkinson's, Alzheimer's and chronic fatigue syndrome.

pelvic inflammatory disease (PID) – Inflammation in the pelvis, often caused by STDs or infection.

pre-implantation genetic diagnosis (PGD) – The genetic investigation of hereditary disorders in an embryo before implantation into the uterus.

polycystic ovary syndrome (PCOS) – Hormone-related condition which causes small, underdeveloped follicles to grow on the ovaries. If left unmanaged, it can cause problems with fertility, as ovulation is less likely to occur.

post-coital test – Test to ensure the sperm is getting through the cervix, which is also used to check for hostile mucus, signs of infection or acidity, altered cervical mucus (too thick), and antibodies which may attack the sperm.

premature ovarian failure – Cessation of ovulation, otherwise known as early menopause.

progesterone – Hormone secreted by the corpus luteum of the ovary after ovulation.

prolactin – Hormone produced by the pituitary gland, the level of which may affect ovulation.

prostatitis – Infection or inflammation of the prostate gland. May cause poor sperm count.

reproductive immunology – Field of medicine specializing in the relationship between the immune system and fertility and pregnancy.

secondary infertility – The inability to conceive or carry a pregnancy to term after having previously had a successful pregnancy.

semen analysis – Evaluation of the number and quality of sperm and how well they move (motility and morphology).

sexually transmitted diseases (STDs) – Often the cause of pelvic inflammatory disease, which can contribute to fertility problems.

sharp curettage – Surgical procedure in which the cervix is expanded using a dilator and the uterine lining scraped with a curette.

sperm freezing – When semen is ejaculated or retrieved and frozen for IVF or future use.

Tamoxifen – Drug commonly used in cancer treatment, and also in fertility treatment when there are ovulation problems, as it inhibits the production of oestrogen.

testosterone – Hormone produced in the male testicles.

thrombophilia – Excessive blood-clotting condition.

varicocele – Enlargement of small veins under one or both testicles.

vasectomy – Surgical procedure for male sterilization.

vitrification – Fast freezing process for eggs.

xenoestrogens – Compounds found in things like insecticides and pesticides that mimic oestrogen in the body and so can disrupt hormonal balance.

APPENDIX III
COMPLEMENTARY TREATMENTS

Acupressure

Acupressure is a simplified version of shiatsu, which is similar in theory to acupuncture, but uses the application of pressure to specific points and channels instead of needles, using thumbs, elbows, forearms and even knees. You can learn how to use acupressure on yourself, as part of a massage routine or to treat specific conditions like headaches or period pains.

Acupuncture

Acupuncture has been used in the Far East to restore, promote and maintain good health for over 2,500 years. Acupuncture is rooted in the Daoist philosophy of change, growth, balance and harmony. Today, 2.3 million acupuncture treatments are carried out each year by acupuncturists registered with the British Acupuncture Council, and the therapy is widely accepted as an effective solution for a huge array of illnesses and symptoms. There are a number of studies which support the positive role acupuncture may have to play in subfertility (see page 7).

In a patient's first acupuncture treatment, the practitioner will take a full medical case history, including past health background and details about the current condition. Once the patient is settled on the treatment couch, a practitioner will carry out pulse-taking on each wrist and examine the patient's tongue. The practitioner will then make a diagnosis and put together a treatment plan, which may include lifestyle and dietary advice as well as acupuncture.

During a typical treatment, practitioners use very fine single-use disposable needles – the needles are as fine as a human hair, nothing like those used for an injection or to take blood. Most people find acupuncture to be very relaxing. My patients often describe the needle sensation as a tingling or dull ache. Some say they don't feel a thing; many even fall asleep during their treatment.

Aromatherapy and massage

Aromatherapy and massage use essential oils to relieve and release emotional or mental stresses and physical strains. Specific oils are used for certain uses, so lavender is well known for its relaxing properties, while citrus oils like grapefruit are used to energize.

Colonic irrigation

Colonic irrigation is a detoxification technique which uses water to cleanse the bowel. It can be helpful for some digestive issues and for conditions such as endometriosis, as well as for general cleansing of your system.

Counselling

Counselling, through charities like Relate, for example, can be very helpful for some couples along the fertility journey. The mind plays such an important part in fertility, and fertility can place extra pressures on relationships and individuals.

Chinese herbal medicine

I work closely with Chinese herbal medicine specialist Michael McIntyre (see Resources). According to Michael, in treating infertility, Chinese herbal treatment seeks to normalize menstrual flow (which ideally should be bright red, without clots, free of spotting or pain) and the cycle, which should approximate to the lunar cycle of 28 days. To achieve this, the practitioner may prescribe a combination of herbs that, according to need, warm or cool the uterus, regularize digestion, calm the Heart spirit, invigorate the flow of Qi (vital energy) and Blood and/or resolve phlegm and Dampness. In addition, herbs are used to balance the activity of the internal organs, particularly the kidney, which in Chinese medicine includes many of the functions of the female hormones oestrogen and progesterone, as well as the pituitary gland (which produces FSH and LH). In addition, herbal remedies can be used to treat conditions that may affect fertility, such as PCOS and endometriosis.[76] Herbs can also often be used to improve male subfertility.

Herb teas often taste strange, but one soon gets used to taking them. The usual length of treatment is three to six months, during which time most herbalists will be more than willing to work alongside a conventional gynaecologist and fit in with assisted reproductive technology (ART). As these herbs have been in use for millennia, they can be considered safe for use in these circumstances. A limited amount of medical research is available to support the herbal treatment of subfertility, but it is encouraging.[77]

Nutrition

Nutrition is crucial for many women when it comes to nourishing and preserving fertility, and also for helping to address many specific conditions associated with fertility, like PCOS, endometriosis and thyroid problems. I am not a qualified nutritionist, but diet is an important part of Chinese medicine. I have asked nutritionist Henrietta Norton to contribute specifically to key aspects of nutrition and fertility throughout the book.

Reflexology

Reflexology applies touch to points on the feet or hands to treat specific parts of the body, for example strengthening digestion or relieving tense and sore shoulders. It can be relaxing and very effective, and if you can't cope with the thought of needles, this might be a good alternative. Like acupuncture, it is based on releasing blocked-energy pathways. It isn't actually known where it originated – some say Egypt, while others say India, China or South America.

REFERENCES

1. Robinson, K. and Hickenbottom, T. 2003. Acupuncture has numerous potential fertility-boosting benefits according to New York Weill Cornell physician-scientists. Cornell University News Service. Available at www.news.cornell.edu/releases/April03/fertility.html.

2. Ng, E. H., So, W. S., Gao, J., Wong, Y. Y. and Ho, P. C. 2008. The role of acupuncture in the management of subfertility. *Fertility and Sterility*, 90 (1): 1–13. Review examining the use of acupuncture in the management of subfertility. Suggests that the positive effects of acupuncture in the treatment of subfertility may be related to central sympathetic inhibition by the endorphin system, the change in uterine blood flow and motility, and stress reduction, and may help restore ovulation in patients with PCOS.

3. Huang, S. T. and Chen, A. P. 2008. Traditional Chinese medicine and infertility. *Current Opinion in Obstetrics and Gynecology*, 20 (3): 211–15. Review examining the use of traditional Chinese medicine in the treatment of infertility. Reports on studies that show acupuncture can regulate gonadotropin-releasing hormone (GnRH) to induce ovulation, improve uterine blood flow and benefit patients with infertility resulting from PCOS, anxiety, stress and immunological disorders.

4. Stener-Victorin, E. and Humaidan, P. 2006. Use of acupuncture in female infertility and a summary of recent acupuncture studies related to embryo transfer. *Acupuncture in Medicine*, 24 (4): 157–63. Review examining clinical and experimental data on the effects of acupuncture on uterine and ovarian blood flow, and on endocrine and metabolic disturbances such as PCOS.

5. Paulus, W., Zhang, M., Strehler, E., et al. 2002. Influence of acupuncture on the pregnancy rate in patients who undergo assisted reproductive therapy. *Fertility and Sterility*, 77 (4), 721–4.

6. Stener-Victorin, E. and Humaidan, P. 2006. Use of acupuncture in female infertility and a summary of recent acupuncture studies related to embryo transfer. *Acupuncture in Medicine*, 24 (4), 157–63.

7. Manheimer, E. et al. 2008. Effects of acupuncture on rates of pregnancy and live birth among women undergoing IVF: systematic review and meta-analysis. *British Medical Journal*, 336 (7743): 545–9. The reviewers concluded that acupuncture given with embryo transfer improves rates of pregnancy and live birth among women undergoing IVF.

8. Mo, X., Li, D., Pu, Y. et al. 1993. Clinical studies on the mechanism for acupuncture stimulation of ovulation. *Journal of Traditional Chinese Medicine*, 13 (2), 115–19.

9. Maughan, Toni A. and Zhai, Xiao-Ping. 2012. The Acupuncture Treatment of Infertility – with Particular Reference to Egg Quality and Endometrial Receptiveness. *Journal of Chinese Medicine*, 98, 13–21.

10. Chen, B.Y. 1997. Acupuncture Normalizes Dysfunction of Hypothalamic-Pituitary –Ovarian Axis. *Acupuncture and Electro-Therapeutics Research*, 22, 97–108.

11. Bentzen, J. G., et al. 2012. Maternal menopause as a predictor of anti-Müllerian hormone level and antral follicle count in daughters during reproductive age. *Human Reproduction*. Available at http://www.medpagetoday.com/upload/2012/11/7/Hum.%20Reprod.-2012-Bentzen-humrep-des356.pdf.

12. Barbieri, R. 2001. The initial fertility consultation: recommendations concerning cigarette smoking, body mass index, and alcohol and caffeine consumption. *American Journal of Obstetrics and Gynecology*, 185: 1168–73.

13. Augood, C., et al. 1998. Smoking and female infertility: a systematic review and meta-analysis. *Human Reproduction*, 13: 1532–9.

14. Wasser, S. K., Sewall, G. and Soules, M. R. 1993. Psychosocial stress as a cause of infertility. *Fertility and Sterility*, 59 (3): 685–9.

15. Deadman, Peter. 2005. How to be Healthy: Traditional Chinese Health Preservation Teachings and Modern Research. *Journal of Chinese Medicine*, 78, 41–48.

16. Zama, A. M., Uzumcu, M. 2010. Epigenetic effects of endocrine-disrupting chemicals on female reproduction: an ovarian perspective. *Front Neuroendoceinol.* 31: 420–39.

17. Gandolfi, F., Pocar, P., Brevini, T.A.L., Fischer, B. 2002. Impact of endocrine disrupters on ovarian function and embryonic development. *Domestic Animal Endocrinology.* 40: 291–99. 16.

18. Meldrum, D.R. 1993. Female reproductive aging: ovarian and uterine factors. *Fertility and Sterility*, 59: 1–5.

19. Krisher, Rebecca L. 2013. In Vivo and In Vitro Environmental Effects on Mammalian Oocyte Quality. National Foundation for Fertility Research. *Animal Biosciences*.

20. Barad et al. 2009. *Fertility and Sterility*, 91(4): 1553–5.

21. Weghofer et al. 2011. *Human Reproduction*, 26 (7): 1905–9).

22. There is a study currently underway (see http://clinicaltrials.gov/ct2/show/NCT00878124) to assess CoEnzyme Q10 and response to fertility drugs for follicle growth stimulation. The results have not yet been published.

23. Wiser, A. et al. 2010. Addition of DHEA for poor-responder patients before and during IVF treatment improves the pregnancy rate. A randomized prospective study. *Human Reproduction*, 25: 2496–500.

24. Gleicher, N. et al. 2010. Improvement in diminished ovarian reserve after DHEA supplementation. *Reproductive BioMedicine Online*, 21: 360–5.

25. D. S. Khalsa, M.D. and C. Stauth. *Meditation as Medicine.* Atria, 2002. Meditating 45-year-old women and men have on average, respectively, 47 per cent and 23 per cent more DHEA (the youth-related hormone) than non-meditators, which helps decrease stress, heighten memory, preserve sexual function, and control weight.

26. Bentov, Y. and Casper, R. F. 2013. The aging oocyte – can mitochondrial function be improved? *Fertility and Sterility*, 99: 18–22.

27. Nehra, D. et al. 2012. Prolonging the female reproductive lifespan and improving egg quality with dietary omega-3 fatty acids. *Aging Cell*, 11 (6): 1046–54.

28. Veleva, Z., et al. High and low BMI increase the risk of miscarriage after IVF/ICSI and FET. *Human Reproduction*. Available at http://humrep.oxfordjournals.org/content/23/4/878.short.

29. Frisch, Rose E. 2003. *Female Fertility and the Body Fat Connection.* Chicago: University of Chicago Press.

30. Bellver, J., Ayllón, Y., Ferrando, M., Melo, M., Goyri, E., et al. 2010. Female obesity impairs in vitro fertilization outcome without affecting embryo quality. *Fertility and Sterility*, 93: 447–54.

31. Clark, A., et al. 1998. Weight loss in obese infertile women results in improvement in reproductive outcome for all forms of fertility treatment. *Human Reproduction*, 13: 1505.

32. Boland, M. P., Lonergan, P., O'Callaghan, D. 2001. Effects of nutrition on endocrine parameters, ovarian physiology, and oocyte and embryo development. *Theriogenology* 55: 1323–40.

33. Zijlistra, F. J. et al. 2003. Anti-inflammatory actions of acupuncture. *Mediators of Inflammation*, 12: 59–69. Review article that discusses the anti-inflammatory action of, and promotion of blood circulation by, acupuncture.

34. Kunzle, R. et al. 2003. Semen quality of male smokers and nonsmokers in infertile couples. *Fertility and Sterility*, 79: 287–91.

35. Vaamonde, D., da Silva-Grigoletto, M. E., Garcia-Manso, J. M., Barrera, N., Vaamonde-Lemos, R. 2012. Physically active men show better semen parameters and hormone values than sedentary men. *European Journal of Applied Physiology*, 112: 3267–73.

36. Cherry, N. et al. 2001. Occupational exposure to solvents and male infertility. *Occupational and Environmental Medicine*, 58: 635–40.

37. Tremelien, K. Oxidative stress and male infertility: a clinical perspective. 2008. *Human Reproduction Update*, 14: 243–58.

38. Kefer, J. C. et al. 2009. Role of antioxidants in the treatment of male infertility. Intro *Journal of Urology*, 16 (5): 449–57.

39. Afeiche, Myriam. 2012. Paper presented at the American Society for Reproductive Medicine's (ASRM) annual conference in California.

40. Attaman, J. A., Toth, T. L., Furtado, J., Campos, H., Hauser, R., Chavaro, J.E. 2012. Dietary fat and semen quality among men attending a fertility clinic. *Human Reproduction*, 2: 1474–86.

41. de la Rochebrochard, E., de Mouzon, J., Thonneau, P. 2010. Fathers over 40 and increased failure to conceive: the lessons of in vitro fertilization in France. *Fertility and Sterility*, 93: 1228–33.

42. Jensen, T., et al. 2004. Body mass index in relation to semen quality and reproductive hormones among 1,558 Danish men. *Fertility and Sterility*, 11; 82: 863–70. 32.

43. Crimmel, A. S. et al. 2001. Withered Yang: a review of traditional Chinese medical treatment of male infertility and erectile dysfunction. *Journal of Andrology*, 22: 173–82. A review discussing the clinical evidence that suggests acupuncture has a regulatory effect on circulatory, endocrine and nervous systems, which may be beneficial in the treatment of male infertility by improving sperm maturation in the epididymis, increasing testosterone levels, and reducing liquid peroxidation of sperm.

44. The Nurses' Health Study.

45. Te Morenga, L. et al. 2013. Dietary sugars and body weight: systematic review and meta-analyses of randomised controlled trials and cohort studies. *British Medical Journal*, 346: e7492.

46. Alberts, H. J., Thewissen, R. and Raes, L. 2012. Dealing with problematic eating

behaviour. The effects of a mindfulness-based intervention on eating behaviour, food cravings, dichotomous thinking and body image concern. *Journal of Nutrition Education and Behavior*, 44 (1): 22–8.

47. Lerchbaum, E., Obermayer-Pietsch, B. M. 2012. Vitamin D and fertility: a systematic review. *European Journal of Endocrinology*. Published online 24 January 2012.

48. Dennis, Nicola A. et al. The level of serum anti-Mullerian hormone correlates with vitamin D status in men and women but not in boys. *The Journal of Clinical Endocrinology and Metabolism*. 04/2012; 97(7):2450-5. DOI:10.1210/ic.2012-1213.

49. Ignarro, L. J., Balestrieri, M., Napoli, C. 2007. Nutrition, physical activity and cardiovascular disease: an update. *Cardiovascular Research*, 73: 326–40.

50. Gudmundsdottir, S. et al. Physical activity and fertility in women: the North-Trondelag Health Study. *Human Reproduction*, vol. 24, 12, 3196–204. New research from the Norwegian University of Science and Technology (NTNU) shows that the body may not have enough energy to support both hard workouts and getting pregnant.

51. Wang, J. Z. et al. 2009. Effects of heat stress during in vitro maturation on cytoplasmic versus nuclear components of mouse oocytes. *Reproduction*, 137: 181–89.

52. Fisher, Helen and J. Anderson Thompson, Jr, 'Sex, sexuality, and serotonin: do sexual side effects of most antidepressants jeopardise romantic love and marriage?' paper delivered at American Psychiatric Association Annual Meeting, 1 May 2004.

53. Yoon, H., Chung, W. S., Park, Y. Y. and Cho, I. H. 2005. Effects of stress on female rats' sexual function. *International Journal of Impotence Research*, vol.17, no. I, 33–8.

54. George Preti and Charles Wysocki, cited in 'Pheromones in male perspiration reduce women's tension, alter hormone response that regulates menstrual cycle', *Penn News*, 14 March 2003.

55. Sharot, T. 2012. *The Optimism Bias*. London: Vintage.

56. Wood, Virginia. 1999. Infertility and the use of Basal Body Temperature. *Journal of Chinese Medicine*, 61, 33–41.

57. Witt et al. 2008. Acupuncture and Tens machines are effective in managing period pain. *American Journal of Obstetrics and Gynaecology*, 198: 166 e1–166.e8.

58. Al-Katanani, Y. M., Paula-Lopes, F. F., Hansen, P. J. 2002. Effects of season and exposure to heat stress oocyte competence in Holstein cows. *J. Dairy Science* 85: 390–96.

59. Kyama, C. et al. 2003. Potential involvement of the immune system in the development of endometriosis. *Reproductive Biology and Endocrinology*, 1: 123.

60. Lundeberg, T. and Lund, I. 2008. Is there a role for acupuncture in endometriosis pain, or endometrialgia? *Acupuncture and Medicine*, 26 (2): 94–110.

61. Lim, C. E. and Wong, W. S. 2010. Current evidence of acupuncture on polycystic ovarian syndrome. *Gynecological Endocrinology*. PCOS clinical studies show that acupuncture significantly increases beta-endorphin levels for up to 24 hours and may have regulatory effects on FSH, LH and androgen via the hypothalamic-pituitary–adrenal axis. Acupuncture is a safe and effective treatment for PCOS without the adverse effects of pharmacological interventions. It may act by increasing blood flow to the ovaries, reducing ovarian volume and the number of ovarian cysts, controlling hyperglycaemia, reducing cortisol levels and assisting in weight loss and anorexia.

62. Stener-Victorin, E. et al. 2008. Acupuncture in polycystic ovary syndrome: current experimental and clinical evidence. *Journal of Neuroendocrinology*, 20 (3): 290–8. Review examining the etiology and pathogenesis of polycystic ovary syndrome (PCOS) and evaluating the use of acupuncture to prevent and reduce symptoms related with PCOS. It concludes that acupuncture can affect PCOS via modulation of the sympathetic nervous system, endocrine and neuroendocrine systems, and suggests that acupuncture can exert long-lasting beneficial effects on metabolic and endocrine systems and ovulation.

63. Arojoki, M. et al. 2000. Hypothyroidism among infertile women in Finland. *Gynaecological Endocrinology*, 14: 127–31. Undiagnosed hypothyroidism is relatively common in infertile women.

64. Veleva et al. 2007. The extremes of BMI are also associated with an increased risk of miscarriage, both in natural pregnancies and after fertility treatment. http://humrep.oxfordjournals.org/content/23/4/878.short).

65. www.hfea.gov.uk

66. Jadeon, J.E., Ben-ami, N., Haddad, S., Radin, O., Bar-ami, S., Younis, J. S. 2012. Prospective evaluation of early follicular ovarian stromal blood flow in infertile women undergoing IVF-ET treatment. *Gynecological Endocrinology*, 28: 356–9.

67. Ried, K. and Stuart, K. 2011. Efficacy of traditional Chinese herbal medicine in the management of female infertility: A systematic review. *Complementary Therapies in Medicine*, 19 (6): 319–31.

68. In a review in the October 2012 edition of *Reproductive BioMedicine Online*, the team from Guy's and St Thomas' found that the simple procedure of endometrial scratching may increase the chance of IVF success.

69. Buckingham, K. L. and Chamley, L. W. 2009. A critical assessment of the role of antiphospholipid antibodies in infertility. *Journal of Reproductive Immunology*, 80: 132–45.

70. Hu, Y. et al. 1999. Maximizing pregnancy rates and limiting higher-order multiple conceptions by determining the optimal number of embryos to transfer based on quality. *Fertility and Sterility*, 4: 650–7.

71. Maheshwari, A. and Bhattacharya, S. 2013. Elective frozen replacement cycles for all: ready for prime time? *Human Reproduction*, 28 (1): 6–9.

72. Davies et al. 2012. Reproductive technologies and the risk of birth defects. *New England Journal of Medicine*, 10. 366 (19): 1803–13).

73. Wen et al.

74. Ola, B. et al. 2001. Should ICSI be the treatment of choice for all cases of in-vitro conception? *Human Reproduction*, 16: 2485–90.

75. Borini, A. et al. 2009. Comparison of IVF and ICSI when only few oocytes are available for insemination. *Reproductive BioMedicine Online*, 19: 270–5.

76. Flower, A., Liu, J. P., Lewith, G., Little, P. and Li, Q. 2012. Chinese herbal medicine for endometriosis. *Cochrane Database of Systematic Reviews*. 16, (5): CD006568. Review.

77. Ried, K. and Stuart, K. 2011. Efficacy of Traditional Chinese Herbal Medicine in the management of female infertility: a systematic review. *Complementary Therapies in Medicine*, 19 (6): 319–31.

RESOURCES

Useful contacts

Emma Cannon Clinics
Appointments: 07531 916 121
emma@emmacannon.co.uk
www.emmacannon.co.uk

Grace Medical
11a West Halkin Street
London SW1X 8JL

and

The Lister
Chelsea Outpatient Centre
280 Kings Road
London SW3 5AW

Contributors

Adrian Lower
Adrian Lower is a consultant gynaecologist and minimal access surgeon based at the Princess Grace Hospital, London. He is an expert in the management of a number of key gynaecological conditions which affect fertility, including uterine fibroids, Asherman's syndrome and endometriosis. He also acts as an independent fertility specialist, preparing and managing assisted conception cycles.
www.adrianlower.com

Michael Dooley
Michael Dooley is a consultant gynaecologist and a Fellow of the Royal College of Obstetricians and Gynaecologists.
The Lister

Chelsea Outpatient Centre
280 Kings Road
London SW3 5AW
www.mdooley.co.uk

James Nicopoullos
Consultant gynaecologist at the Lister.
www.ivf.org.uk

Bill Smith
Head of ultrasound, Clinical Diagnostic Services.
info@clinicaldiagnostics.co.uk

Tim Weeks
Women's health and fitness specialist.
www.timweeks.co.uk

Henrietta Norton
Nutritionist, specializing in women's health.
www.henriettanorton.com

Uma Dinsmore-Tuli
Uma Dinsmore-Tuli has developed yoga courses specially designed to support
women's health and healing.
www.wombyoga.org
www.yonishakti.co

Fiona Arrigo
Life teacher and psychotherapist.
www.thearrigoprogramme.com

Adriana Giotta
Counsellor and specialist in women's body issues.
www.linkedin.com/in/adrianagiotta

Shideh Pouria
A medical doctor specializing in environmental and nutritional medicine.
www.gracebelgravia.com

Helpful associations and websites

International Asherman's Association
An organization whose mission is to preserve women's fertility and reproductive health by creating international awareness of intrauterine adhesions
(Asherman's syndrome), an acquired condition which can cause infertility,
characterized by the formation of adhesions (scar tissue) inside the uterus.
www.ashermans.org

Journal of Chinese Medicine
This journal was established in 1979 by Peter Deadman and has been
published continuously ever since. It has played a vital role in raising the
standards of education and practice in Chinese medicine throughout the
English-speaking world. Since 2001, the journal website has been offering
the very best Chinese medicine books for sale and in March 2005 greatly
expanded the range of online products to include herbs, acupuncture supplies
and specialist teas.
www.jcm.co.uk/tea-shop

Fertility UK
Health professionals who specialize in fertility awareness.
www.fertilityuk.org

Duo Fertility
Fertility monitoring service.
http://www.duofertility.com

www.fertilityfriend.com; www.fertilityplus.org
Websites to help with charting your menstrual cycle.

www.lifechoicesandfertility.com
A website to provide couples with up-to-date information, including
descriptions of reseach and units.

Smokefree
NHS advice for quitting smoking.
www.smokefree.nhs.uk

Overeaters Anonymous
Local meetings for those struggling with food issues.
www.oagb.org.uk

Alcoholics Anonymous
A fellowship of men and women who share their experience and strength with each other in the hope that they may solve their common problem and help others to recover from alcoholism.
www.alcoholics-anonymous.org.uk

Neal's Yard Remedies
Stockists of herbs and natural remedies.
www.nealsyardremedies.com

Infertility Network UK
The leading national infertility charity, IN UK works to ensure anyone trying to conceive who needs support, information or advice for their fertility or infertility can find it easily and in one place. IN UK leads the campaign for fair and equitable access to NHS-funded treatment.
www.infertilitynetworkuk.com

Human Fertilization and Embryology Authority
The UK's independent regulator, overseeing the use of gametes and embryos in fertility treatment and research.
www.hfea.gov.uk

Royal College of Obstetricians and Gynaecologists
The RCOG encourages the study and advancement of the science and practice of obstetrics and gynaecology through postgraduate medical education and training development and the publication of clinical guidelines, and reports on aspects of the speciality and service provision.
www.rcog.org.uk

Immunological testing
If you want to read arguments both for and against immunological testing, research is available on the following websites:

Against:
rcog.org.uk/womens-health/clinical-guidance/immunological-testing-and-interventions-reproductive-failure
hfea.gov.uk/fertility-treatment-options-reproductive-immunology.html
For:
www.repro-med.net
www.centerforhumanreprod.com

National Institute for Clinical Excellence
www.nice.org.uk

British Acupuncture Council
The UK's main regulatory body for the practice of traditional acupuncture.
www.acupuncture.org.uk

Meridian Press
For more information about Chinese dietary therapy.
www.meridianpress.net

Sitaram Yoga
Established in 1998, Sitaram Yoga offers a unique programme of yoga, yoga therapy and hypnosis.
www.sitaram.org

Register of Chinese Herbal Medicine
The Register of Chinese Herbal Medicine was set up in 1987 to regulate the practice of Chinese herbal medicine (CHM) in the UK and has over 450 members.
www.rchm.co.uk

British Agency for Fostering and Adoption
www.baaf.org.uk

British Association for Counselling and Psychotherapy
www.bacp.co.uk

Trying for Number Two
Blog about the experience of secondary infertility.
http://tryingfornumbertwo.blogspot.com

One at a Time
A professionally led website aimed at reducing the risk of multiple pregnancies from fertility treatment.
www.oneatatime.org.uk

The Multiple Births Foundation
An independent charity based at Queen Charlotte's and Chelsea Hospital in London, aiming to improve the care and support of multiple birth families.
www.multiplebirths.org.uk

Meditation Foundation
A Department of Health-supported social enterprise offering simple, modern, evidence-based, non-religious meditation and mindfulness courses and retreats.
www.meditationfoundation.org

Andrology Solutions
An independent, scientist-led, HFEA-licensed fertility clinic that specializes solely in male-related fertility issues.
www.andrologysolutions.co.uk

Center for Human Reproduction
For lots more information on DHEA visit this website and go to the Top Treatments section.
www.centerforhumanreprod.com

SUGGESTED READING

Alan E. Beer MD, *Is Your Body Baby-Friendly?*, AJR Publishing LLC, 2006.

Harriet Beinfield and Erfrem Korngold, *Between Heaven and Earth*, Ballantine Books, 1991.

Tara Bennett-Goleman, *Emotional Alchemy*, Harmony Books, 2001.

Emma Cannon, *You and Your Bump*, Macmillan, 2011.

Emma Cannon, *The Baby-Making Bible*, Macmillan, 2012.

Lorraine Clissold, *Why the Chinese Don't Count Calories*, Constable, 2008.

Peter Deadman. 2005. How to be Healthy: Traditional Chinese Health Preservation Teachings and Modern Research. *Journal of Chinese Medicine*, 78: 41–49.

Rose Elliot, *The Kitchen Pharmacy*, Orion, 1998.

M. Esther Harding, *The Way of All Women*, Shambhala, 1990.

Rick Gallop, *The G.I. Diet*, Virgin Books, 2005.

Paul Gilbert, *The Compassionate Mind*, Constable, 2009.

Marilyn Glenville, *Natural Solutions to PCOS*, Macmillan, 2012.

David R. Hamilton, *Why Kindness is Good For You*, Hay House, 2010.

Benjamin Hoff, *The Tao of Pooh*, Methuen Young Books, 2002.

Gab Kovacs (ed.), *How to Improve Your ART Success Rates*, Cambridge University Press, 2011.

Daverick Leggett, *Helping Ourselves: A Guide to Traditional Chinese Food Energetics*, Meridian Press, 1994.

Jane Lyttleton, *Treatment of Infertility with Chinese Medicine*, Churchill Livingstone, 2004.

Gil Mor, *The Immunology of Pregnancy*, Landes Bioscience, 2006.

Brigid Moss, *IVF: An Emotional Companion*, Collins, 2011.

Christiane Northrup MD, *Women's Bodies, Women's Wisdom*, 2006.

Christiane Northrup MD and Kristina Tracy, *Beautiful Girl*, Hay House, 2012.

Henrietta Norton, *Take Control of Your Endometriosis*, Kyle Books, 2012.

Yotam Ottolenghi, *Plenty*, Ebury Press, 2010.

Yotam Ottolenghi, *Jerusalem*, Ebury Press, 2012.

Don Miguel Ruiz, *The Four Agreements*, Amber-Allen Publishing, 1997.

T. W. Sadler, *Langman's Medical Embryology*, Wolters Kluwer, 1999.

Tali Sharot, *The Optimism Bias*, Vintage, 2012.

John Shi et al., *Functional Foods of the East*, CRC Press, 2010.

Naomi Wolf, *Vagina*, Virago, 2013.

INDEX